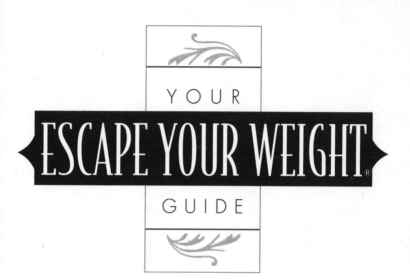

YOUR

# ESCAPE YOUR WEIGHT

GUIDE

# DR. EDWARD JACKOWSKI

◆

THOMAS DUNNE BOOKS

St. Martin's Griffin

New York

ALSO BY EDWARD JACKOWSKI, Ph.D.

*Escape Your Shape*

*Hold It! You're Exercising Wrong*

THOMAS DUNNE BOOKS.
An imprint of St. Martin's Press.

www.stmartins.com

Design by Patrice Sheridan

ISBN 0-312-32050-7

First Edition: April 2003

10  9  8  7  6  5  4  3  2  1

# Contents

It Doesn't Matter What Plan of Action You Choose

to Lose Weight as Long as the Plan You've Chosen Is Practical

and One That You Can Adhere to Without Deviating!

# How to Use Your Escape Your Weight Guide

Not everyone enjoys dieting nor can they stick to extreme diets for long periods of time without resorting back to their former eating patterns in one form or another. On the other hand, there are also those who loathe exercise and cannot and will not work out 5, 6 or 7 days a week no matter what you tell them or incentives you throw at them. During our childhood, adolescence, young adulthood and as an adult, we have all formed certain patterns, likes and dislikes regarding our eating and exercise habits. When it comes to weight loss, one thing is certain: we need to create a caloric deficit in order to lose weight. To be more successful at it long-term, the amount of calories we expend at the end of any given day *must* be greater than the amount of calories we've consumed for that particular day—on a consistent basis.

There are many techniques that we can employ in order for this to occur. *Your Escape Your Weight Guide* is designed for you to choose the weight loss path that puts the least amount of stress on your mind and body. In other words, if you are used to or prefer to diet more than exercise in order to achieve weight loss, then choose that plan and stick to it. Or, perhaps you'd rather exercise a bit more rather than diet to lose weight, choose that particular plan and you'll be successful as well. What's important is that whichever approach you choose, you follow the procedures for dieting and/or exercise *precisely* as outlined, thus insuring that you'll attain permanent weight loss.

Each weight loss category is broken down with a precise diet and exercise regimen for you to follow. Based on your approach that you choose, make sure that you are only taking in the allotted amount of calories for the day matched up with the exercise regimen and frequency needed for you to lose and keep losing weight until you get to your desired weight. Once you've chosen your pill you now can follow the diet and exercise routine that you feel most comfortable with to propel you towards your weight loss goals. Good luck!

# ONE

# Introduction to Approaches

I'm sure you've heard the phrase, "you can't have it all." It's true, and especially when it comes to losing weight. There are only three effective ways to lose weight through natural means: a) severely restrict your caloric intake with a little exercise sprinkled in (**Restrictive**); b) work out like a fiend while watching your diet only a little bit (**Excessive**); and c) eat sensibly most of the time coupled with regular exercise (**Equilibrium**). These are your options and you'll have to choose one in order to lose and keep weight off. The path (approach) you choose has mostly to do with your current views and feelings towards diet and exercise that have been influenced since childhood. For instance, some of you may find that severely restricting your caloric intake is less shocking to you both mentally and physically because in the past, you were *initially* successful with weight loss. Or, you don't want to "diet" and would rather exercise more so that you feel that you're not depriving yourself. And lastly, you don't mind watching and monitoring your food intake (most of the time) coupled with exercising on a regular basis.

Whichever approach you decide to take, it's important to

note that **each of the three** methods and approaches involve *both* a reduction in caloric intake *and* an exercise component. Both are crucial for you to lose weight, be fit, raise your Basal Metabolic Rate (BMR), which is the ability to burn calories during resting state, and maintain weight loss. All you need to do is choose the path of least resistance and follow the recommended diet and exercise frequency from *Your Escape Your Weight Guide*, and you're on your way to becoming successful with permanent weight loss. Please note that all thr_e approaches will yield results *if, and only if,* you follow the guidelines outlined in detail for each of the three approaches. For instance, if you choose the **Restrictive** approach, you cannot arbitrarily decide to all of a sudden eat whatever you wish or not exercise at all and fantasize that you'll lose weight. All three approaches are designed so that you get to choose what method you will feel most comfortable with to help you achieve long-term weight loss.

Below you'll find certain characteristics, helpful tips and guidelines to follow for all three approaches. Once you've reviewed them all, then choose the eating plan and exercise routine that is outlined and detailed for each approach and weight loss category.

### ✦ RESTRICTIVE: ⊘

Quite simply, the thought of exercising is not exactly a turn-on to you and given the choice (which you now have), you would rather *restrict* the total amount of calories taken in over the course of a day, week or month versus exercising 5 days per week in order to create a deficit of calories necessary to lose weight. "Dieting" is not as shocking to your system and is less stressful to you than going to the gym day-in and day-out. As you can see from the Diet/Exercise Guide (page 4), you only need to work out 2 days a week combined with severely cutting your calories in order to shed those pounds.

## ✦ EXCESSIVE:

You are the type who uses activity/exercise to counter the food you ingest so that you won't gain weight. "Dieting" is a no-no, and there's no way you are going to deprive yourself of your favorite foods. And guess what? You still won't have to deny yourself that pleasure *but* you will have to be conscious of the amount of that favorite food you're eating and start to cut back on the amount you are eating, called *portion control*. In order to be successful at permanent weight loss (see Diet/ Exercise Guide on page 4), you only need to carefully monitor your total caloric intake a few days a week, provided, of course, that you are willing to work out most days of the week.

## ✦ EQUILIBRIUM:

You're the type of person who "exercises" regularly and when you need to, will pay careful attention to your caloric intake. Most of the time, you're pretty good with both eating and exercise and you don't like extreme "dieting" or excessive exercise. You won't "diet" per se on a long-term basis, but just enough in order to lose weight, perhaps because you have a social event coming up or you soon need to put on a slinky dress or bathing suit. Your formula for success (see Diet/Exercise Guide on page 4), involves eating sensibly 5 days per week coupled with moving (exercising, not merely being active) 4–5 days per week in order to achieve your weight loss goals.

## ✦ SUMMARY

Now that you know which approach you're going to enact, all you need to do is be honest with yourself and give 100%.

# ESCAPE YOUR WEIGHT—DIET/EXERCISE GUIDE

| | Diet Frequency: # of days/week (diet needs to be good) | Exercise Frequency: # of Days Need to Exercise | Intensity of Exercise: Low–Moderate–High | Type: Aerobic vs. Anaerobic: Percent Time Spent During 60 Minutes of Exercise |
|---|---|---|---|---|
| Weight Loss 75+ lbs. **Restrictive** | 7 | 2 | Low-Moderate | 80–90% Aerobic 10–20% Anaerobic |
| Weight Loss 75+ lbs. **Excessive** | 2 | 6–7 | Moderate | 80–90% Aerobic 10–20% Anaerobic |
| Weight Loss 75+ lbs. **Equilibrium** | 5 | 4–5 | Moderate | 80–90% Aerobic 10–20% Anaerobic |
| Weight Loss 25–74 lbs. **Restrictive** | 7 | 2 | Moderate | 70% Aerobic 30% Anaerobic |
| Weight Loss 25–74 lbs. **Excessive** | 3 | 6–7 | Moderate | 70% Aerobic 30% Anaerobic |
| Weight Loss 25–74 lbs. **Equilibrium** | 5 | 4–5 | Moderate-high | 70% Aerobic 30% Anaerobic |
| Weight Loss –25 lbs. **Restrictive** | 7 | 2 | Moderate | 60% Aerobic 40% Anaerobic |
| Weight Loss –25 lbs. **Excessive** | 4 | 6–7 | Moderate | 60% Aerobic 40% Anaerobic |
| Weight Loss –25 lbs. **Equilibrium** | 5 | 4–5 | High | 60% Aerobic 40% Anaerobic |

Remember, it doesn't matter which approach you choose as long as you follow the diet plans and exercise prescriptions outlined for each because all three are effective. You do, however, want to eventually gravitate towards **Equilibrium**, because it allows you more room for error *and* over time, you won't have to shock your mind, body and system with either severely restricting your diet or by exercising excessively.

## ◆ EQUIPMENT NEEDED

**DUAL-FOLD EXERCISE MAT**

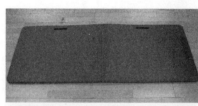

**THE EXUDE SPEED ROPE**

**DUMBBELLS**

**OR**

**AEROBIC TONING BAR**

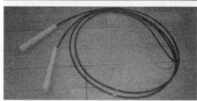

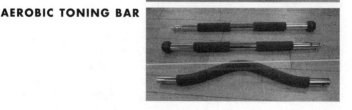

(Optional)
Trampoline
Rebounder

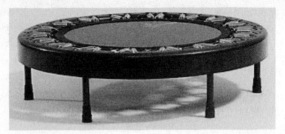

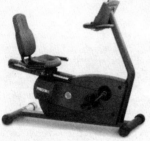

a.

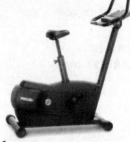

b.

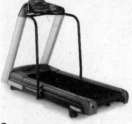

c.

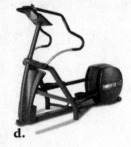

d.

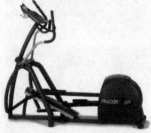

e.

Please select one (or more) of
the following:
a. Recumbent bike
b. Upright bike
c. Treadmill
d. Elliptical
e. Crosstrainer
(Precor® Fitness Equipment)

# ◆ HELPFUL TIPS FOR SUCCESSFUL WEIGHT REDUCTION:

### Keep a Food Journal—Write Down What and When You Eat and Drink in a Day and Why

The journal will help you become aware of what you eat, will increase your control over eating and will help you become aware of your eating patterns—food becomes fattening when it is eaten for entertainment, comfort or stress reduction.

### Become Aware of Meal Timing

Eating earlier in the day prevents you from getting too hungry, losing control, and overeating in the evening.

### Learn Your Calorie Budget

Know how much you can eat and still lose weight so you can be sure to fuel your body with an adequate amount of essential nutrients.

### Eat Slowly

The brain needs about 20 minutes to receive the signal that you've eaten your fill. Practice by putting your fork down between bites and taking pauses throughout the meal.

### Keep Away from Food Sources That Tempt You

Out of sight, out of mind, out of MOUTH! Hide high calorie foods and keep healthy snacks readily available.

### Taste Your Food

Calories should be tasted, not wasted. Do nothing else while eating and really savor your food.

### Stick To Your Shopping List

Always bring a food list when grocery shopping and never shop while hungry!

### Buy Individually Wrapped Packages

Buy your favorite snack foods in individual serving sizes to avoid overeating and further temptation.

### Set Realistic Goals

Weight loss greater than 1% of your body weight for over 2 weeks can be dangerous . . . you can lose muscle, including cardiac muscle. Aim to lose 1–2 pounds per week to ensure you are losing primarily body fat.

## ◆ HIDDEN CALORIE FOODS/FOODS TO AVOID

- Movie theater popcorn—large with butter contains 1640 calories and 126 gm fat (73 gm saturated!)
- Prime rib—16 oz contains 1280 calories and 94 gm fat (52 gm saturated)
- Cheese—1 oz contains 100 calories and 9 gm fat (6 gm saturated)
- Pizza (⅛ pie)—250 calories and 7 gm fat (4 gm saturated)
- General Tso's chicken—1600 calories and 59 gm fat (11 gm saturated)
- Hamburgers—6-oz burger on a bun contains 660 calories and 36 gm fat (17 gm saturated)
- Doughnuts—an old-fashioned cake doughnut contains 250 calories and 15 gm fat (3 gm saturated)
- Cinnamon rolls—670 calories and 34 gm fat (14 gm saturated)
- Croissants—5-oz almond croissant contains 630 calories and 42 gm fat (18 gm saturated)

- French fries—large order contains 500 calories and 28 gm fat (13 gm saturated fat)
- Tortilla chips—typical basket (51 chips) contains 640 calories and 34 gm fat (6 gm saturated)
- Grilled cheese sandwich—500 calories and 33 gm fat (17 gm saturated fat)
- Fettuccine Alfredo—1500 calories and 97 gm fat (48 gm saturated)
- Starbucks white chocolate mocha (made with whole milk)—600 calories and 25 gm fat (15 gm saturated)
- Pancakes with syrup and margarine (3 pancakes with ¼ cup syrup and 1 tbsp margarine)—770 calories and 22 gm fat (9 gm saturated)

TWO

# Diet Plans for Losing 75 Pounds or More

## MEAL PLAN TO LOSE 75 POUNDS OR MORE
*RESTRICTIVE APPROACH*

### 1800 CALORIES PER DAY
(247 gm carbohydrate, 90 gm protein, 50 gm fat)

---

**BREAKFAST** (*600 calories, approx. 82 gm carbohydrate, 30 gm protein, 16 gm fat*):

1. (600 calories, 82 gm carb, 28 gm protein, 15 gm fat)
   2¼ cups whole grain cereal (unsweetened, ready-to-eat cereal)
   1½ cups skim milk
   1¼ cups berries
   12 almonds
   1 hard-boiled egg

2. (600 calories, 79 gm carb, 30 gm protein, 17 gm fat)
   ¾ cup 1% cottage cheese
   1 cup berries
   1 cup melon
   1 cup Grape-Nuts
   12 almonds
   2 slices of whole grain bread
   2 tsp peanut butter

3. (600 calories, 82 gm carb, 29 gm protein, 15 gm fat)
   2 slices of whole grain bread
   1 tbsp peanut butter
   1 apple
   12 oz low-fat yogurt
   $^1/_2$ cup low-fat granola

4. (600 calories, 80 gm carb, 28 gm protein, 15 gm fat)
   2 poached eggs
   2 slices of whole grain bread
   $^3/_4$ cup plain low-fat yogurt
   $1^1/_2$ cups melon
   1 cup mixed berries

5. (600 calories, 78 gm carb, 33 gm protein, 15 gm fat)
   2 cups cooked oatmeal
   12 chopped walnut halves
   1 chopped red delicious apple

$^3/_4$ cup low-fat cottage cheese

6. (600 calories, 80 gm carb, 27 gm protein, 15 gm fat)
   Omelet—2 whole eggs + $^1/_2$ oz of low-fat cheese + $^1/_2$ cup spinach + $^1/_2$ cup chopped tomato
   2 slices of whole grain bread
   1 cup sliced strawberries
   1 sliced kiwi
   1 cup cubed melon

7. (600 calories, 84 gm carb, 30 gm protein, 16 gm fat)
   2 slices of whole grain bread
   2 oz cheese
   $^1/_2$ cup sliced tomato
   $2^1/_2$ cups mixed melon
   1 cup skim milk

**LUNCH** *(600 calories, approx. 82 gm carbohydrate, 30 gm protein, 16 gm fat):*

1. (600 calories, 80 gm carb, 29 gm protein, 15 gm fat)
   2 slices of whole grain bread
   3 oz white meat turkey
   $^1/_4$ avocado
   $^1/_2$ cup sliced tomato/lettuce
   1 cup unsweetened apple sauce with $^1/_4$ cup granola

2. (600 calories, 80 gm carb, 29 gm protein, 15 gm fat)
   1 whole wheat pita
   3 oz chunk white tuna fish

3 tsp mayonnaise
$^1/_2$ cup mixed shredded carrots, lettuce and celery
36 cherries

3. (600 calories, 80 gm carb, 29 gm protein, 15 gm fat)
   3 oz of cold chicken (cut up) mix with 3 tsp mayonnaise
   2 slices of rye bread
   $^1/_2$ cup sliced tomato and lettuce
   1 whole diced mango
   1 cup raspberries

4. (600 calories, 80 gm carb, 35
   gm protein, 15 gm fat)
   Big Salad:
   2 cups mixed greens
   1/2 cup diced carrots
   1/2 cup diced bell peppers
   1/3 cup beans
   3 oz grilled chicken
   4 chopped walnuts
   1 diced apple
   2 tbsp vinaigrette salad dressing
   1 medium nectarine
   6-inch whole wheat pita

5. (600 calories, 85 gm carb, 31
   gm protein, 15 gm fat)
   3 oz lean roast beef
   2 slices rye bread
   1 tsp mayonnaise
   1/2 cup sliced tomato and lettuce
   1/2 cup carrot sticks
   1 1/2 cup fresh pineapple + 1
   cup diced papaya topped
   with 6 slivered almonds

6. (600 calories, 80 gm carb, 30
   gm protein, 15 gm fat)
   3 cups spinach
   1 oz feta cheese
   1 oz firm tofu
   1/2 cup water chestnuts
   1/2 cup snap peas
   1 1/2 cup mandarin oranges
   1 tbsp reduced fat ginger
   salad dressing
   10 whole grain crackers

7. (600 calories, 80 gm carb, 31
   gm protein, 15 gm fat)
   2 slices of whole grain bread
   2 oz white meat turkey
   1 oz low-fat cheese
   2 tsp mayonnaise
   1/2 cup sliced tomato and
   lettuce
   1 1/2 cup mixed fruit salad
   3 whole wheat graham
   crackers

## DINNER *(600 calories, approx. 82 gm carbohydrate, 30 gm protein, 16 gm fat):*

1. (600 calories, 85 gm carb, 28
   gm protein, 15 gm fat)
   2 oz cooked chicken (no skin)
   1 cup brown rice
   1 cup green beans sautéed in
   1 tsp olive oil and 6 slivered
   almonds
   1 cup mixed greens with 1/2
   cup chopped tomatoes and
   1/2 cup chopped peppers
   1 tbsp salad dressing

   1 medium apple

2. (600 calories, 85 gm carb, 26
   gm protein, 16 gm fat)
   2 oz lean cooked roast beef
   2/3 cup brown rice
   1/2 cup carrots
   1/2 cup cauliflower
   2 tsp olive oil
   1 whole grain dinner roll
   1 orange

3. (600 calories, 83 gm carb, 29
   gm protein, 16 gm fat)
   2 oz broiled salmon
   large sweet potato
   1 cup sautéed spinach with
   2 tsp olive oil
   1 cup sliced tomato
   1 1/2 cup diced melon

4. (600 calories, 85 gm carb, 30
   gm protein, 16 gm fat)
   2 oz sautéed shrimp in
   2 tsp. olive oil
   1 1/2 cups whole wheat pasta
   1/2 cup jarred tomato sauce
   1/2 cup artichoke hearts
   1/2 cup spinach
   1 1/4 cups sliced strawberries
   1 sliced fresh peach

5. (600 calories, 80 gm carb, 32
   gm protein, 16 gm fat)
   3 oz baked cod
   1/3 cup cooked whole-wheat
   couscous

2 cups baked winter squash
1 cup mixed greens
(kale, collard and
mustard) sautéed in 3 tsp
olive oil
2 cups cubed papaya

6. (600 calories, 85 gm carb, 27
   gm protein, 16 gm fat)
   2 oz flank steak
   1 cup whole wheat couscous
   2 cups roasted broccoli and
   cauliflower with 2 tsp olive oil
   1 1/2 cup raspberries

7. (500 calories, 83 gm carb, 27
   gm protein, 16 gm fat)
   2 oz BBQ chicken
   1 medium corn on the cob
   1 cup baked beans
   1 1/2 cup cucumber and
   tomato salad tossed with 2
   tbsp olive oil–based dressing
   1/2 cup cubed watermelon

# MEAL PLAN TO LOSE 75 POUNDS OR MORE
*EXCESSIVE APPROACH*

## 2200 CALORIES PER DAY
(274 gm carbohydrate, 98 gm protein, 56 gm fat)

**BREAKFAST** *(600 calories, approx. 82 gm carbohydrate, 30 gm protein, 16 gm fat):*

1. (600 calories, 78 gm carb, 33 gm protein, 15 gm fat)
   2¼ cups whole grain cereal (unsweetened, ready-to-eat cereal)
   1½ cup skim milk
   1¼ cup berries
   12 almonds
   1 hard-boiled egg

2. (600 calories, 79 gm carb, 30 gm protein, 17 gm fat)
   ¾ cup 1% cottage cheese
   1 cup berries
   1 cup melon
   1 cup Grape-Nuts
   12 almonds
   2 slices of whole grain bread
   2 tsp peanut butter

3. (600 calories, 82 gm carb, 29 gm protein, 15 gm fat)
   2 slices of whole grain bread
   1 tsp peanut butter
   1 apple
   12 oz low-fat yogurt
   ½ cup low-fat granola

4. (600 calories, 80 gm carb, 28 gm protein, 15 gm fat)
   2 poached eggs
   2 slices of whole grain bread
   ¾ cup plain low-fat yogurt
   1½ cups melon
   1 cup mixed berries

5. (600 calories, 78 gm carb, 33 gm protein, 15 gm fat)
   2 cups cooked oatmeal
   12 chopped walnut halves
   1 chopped red delicious apple
   ¾ cup low-fat cottage cheese

6. (600 calories, 80 gm carb, 27 gm protein, 15 gm fat)
   Omelet—2 whole eggs + ½ oz of low-fat cheese + ½ cup spinach + ½ cup chopped tomato
   2 slices of whole grain bread
   1 cup sliced strawberries
   1 sliced kiwi
   1 cup cubed melon

7. (600 calories, 84 gm carb, 30 gm protein, 16 gm fat)
   2 slices of whole grain bread
   2 oz cheese
   ½ cup sliced tomato
   2½ cups mixed melon
   1 cup skim milk

**LUNCH** (*600 calories, approx. 82 gm carbohydrate, 30 gm protein, 16 gm fat*):

1. (600 calories, 80 gm carb, 29 gm protein, 15 gm fat)
   2 slices of whole grain bread
   3 oz white meat turkey
   ¼ avocado
   ½ cup sliced tomato and lettuce
   1 cup unsweetened apple sauce with ¼ cup granola

2. (600 calories, 80 gm carb, 29
gm protein, 15 gm fat)
1 whole wheat pita
3 oz chunk white tuna fish
3 tsp mayonnaise
1/2 cup mixed shredded
carrots, lettuce and celery
36 cherries

3. (600 calories, 80 gm carb, 29
gm protein, 15 gm fat)
3 oz of cold chicken (cut up)
mix with 3 tsp mayonnaise
2 slices of rye bread
1/2 cup sliced tomato and lettuce
1 whole diced mango
1 cup raspberries

4. (600 calories, 80 gm carb, 35
gm protein, 15 gm fat)
Big Salad:
2 cups mixed greens
1/2 cup diced carrots
1/2 cup diced bell peppers
1/3 cup beans
3 oz grilled chicken
4 chopped walnuts
1 diced apple
2 tbsp vinaigrette salad dressing
1 medium nectarine
6-inch whole wheat pita

5. (600 calories, 85 gm carb,
31 gm protein, 15 gm fat)

3 oz lean roast beef
2 slices rye bread
1 tsp mayonnaise
1/2 cup sliced tomato and lettuce
1/2 cup carrot sticks
1 1/2 cup fresh pineapple
+ 1 cup diced papaya topped
with 6 slivered almonds

6. (600 calories, 80 gm carb, 30
gm protein, 15 gm fat)
3 cups spinach
1 oz feta cheese
1 oz firm tofu
1/2 cup water chestnuts
1/2 cup snap peas
1 1/2 cup mandarin oranges
1 tbsp reduced fat ginger
salad dressing
10 whole grain crackers

7. (600 calories, 80 gm carb, 31
gm protein, 15 gm fat)
2 slices of whole grain bread
2 oz white meat turkey
1 oz low-fat cheese
2 tsp mayonnaise
1/2 cup sliced tomato and
lettuce
1 1/2 cups mixed fruit salad
3 whole wheat graham
crackers

**DINNER** *(600 calories, approx. 82 gm carbohydrate, 30 gm
protein, 16 gm fat):*

1. (600 calories, 85 gm carb, 28
gm protein, 15 gm fat)

2 oz cooked chicken (no skin)
1 cup brown rice

1 cup green beans sautéed in
1 tsp olive oil and 6 slivered
almonds
1 cup mixed greens with $^1/_2$
cup chopped tomatoes and
$^1/_2$ cup chopped peppers
1 tbsp salad dressing
1 medium apple

2. (600 calories, 85 gm carb, 26
   gm protein, 16 gm fat)
   2 oz lean cooked roast beef
   $^2/_3$ cup brown rice
   $^1/_2$ cup carrots
   $^1/_2$ cup cauliflower
   2 tsp olive oil
   1 whole grain dinner roll
   1 orange

3. (600 calories, 83 gm carb, 29
   gm protein, 16 gm fat)
   2 oz broiled salmon
   large sweet potato
   1 cup sautéed spinach with 2
   tsp olive oil
   1 cup sliced tomato
   $1^1/_2$ cups diced melon

4. (600 calories, 85 gm carb, 30
   gm protein, 16 gm fat)
   2 oz sautéed shrimp in
   2 tsp olive oil
   $1^1/_2$ cups whole wheat pasta
   $^1/_2$ cup tomato sauce

$^1/_2$ cup artichoke hearts
$^1/_2$ cup spinach
$1^1/_4$ cups sliced strawberries
1 sliced fresh peach

5. (600 calories, 80 gm carb, 32
   gm protein, 16 gm fat)
   3 oz baked cod
   $^1/_3$ cup cooked whole wheat
   couscous
   2 cups baked winter squash
   1 cup mixed greens (kale,
   collard and mustard) sautéed
   in 3 tsp olive oil
   2 cups cubed papaya

6. (600 calories, 85 gm carb, 27
   gm protein, 16 gm fat)
   2 oz flank steak
   1 cup whole wheat couscous
   2 cups roasted broccoli and
   cauliflower with 2 tsp olive
   oil
   $1^1/_2$ cups raspberries

7. (500 calories, 83 gm carb, 27
   gm protein, 16 gm fat)
   2 oz BBQ chicken
   1 medium corn on the cob
   1 cup baked beans
   $1^1/_2$ cup cucumber and
   tomato salad tossed with 2
   tbsp olive oil–based dressing
   $^1/_2$ cup cubed watermelon

**CHOOSE TWO SNACKS FROM PAGES 20–21.**

# MEAL PLAN TO LOSE 75 POUNDS OR MORE
*EQUILIBRIUM APPROACH*

## 2000 CALORIES PER DAY
(274 gm carbohydrate, 98 gm protein, 56 gm fat)

---

**BREAKFAST** *(600 calories, approx. 82 gm carbohydrate, 30 gm protein, 16 gm fat):*

1. (600 calories, 82 gm carb, 28 gm protein, 15 gm fat)
$2^1$/4 cups whole grain cereal (unsweetened, ready-to-eat cereal)
$1^1$/2 cup skim milk
$1^1$/4 cup berries
12 almonds
1 hard-boiled egg

2. (600 calories, 79 gm carb, 30 gm protein, 17 gm fat)
$^3$/4 cup 1% cottage cheese
1 cup berries
1 cup melon
1 cup Grape-Nuts
12 almonds
2 slices of whole grain bread
2 tsp peanut butter

3. (600 calories, 82 gm carb, 29 gm protein, 15 gm fat)
2 slices of whole grain bread
1 tbsp peanut butter
1 apple
12 oz low-fat yogurt
$^1$/2 cup low-fat granola

4. (600 calories, 80 gm carb, 28 gm protein, 15 gm fat)
2 poached eggs
2 slices of whole grain bread
$^3$/4 cup plain low-fat yogurt
$1^1$/2 cups melon
1 cup mixed berries

5. (600 calories, 78 gm carb, 33 gm protein, 15 gm fat)
2 cups cooked oatmeal
12 chopped walnut halves
1 chopped red delicious apple
$^3$/4 cup low-fat cottage cheese

6. (600 calories, 80 gm carb, 27 gm protein, 15 gm fat)
Omelet—2 whole eggs + $^1$/2 oz of low-fat cheese + $^1$/2 cup spinach + $^1$/2 cup chopped tomato
2 slices of whole grain bread
1 cup sliced strawberries
1 sliced kiwi
1 cup cubed melon

7. (600 calories, 84 gm carb, 30 gm protein, 16 gm fat)
   2 slices of whole grain bread
   2 oz cheese
   ½ cup sliced tomato
   2½ cups mixed melon
   1 cup skim milk

## LUNCH *(600 calories, approx. 82 gm carbohydrate, 30 gm protein, 16 gm fat):*

1. (600 calories, 80 gm carb, 29 gm protein, 15 gm fat)
   2 slices of whole grain bread
   3 oz white meat turkey
   ¼ avocado
   ½ cup sliced tomato and lettuce
   1 cup unsweetened apple sauce with ¼ cup granola

2. (600 calories, 80 gm carb, 29 gm protein, 15 gm fat)
   1 whole wheat pita
   3 oz chunk white tuna fish
   3 tsp mayonnaise
   ½ cup mixed shredded carrots, lettuce and celery
   36 cherries

3. (600 calories, 80 gm carb, 29 gm protein, 15 gm fat)
   3 oz of cold chicken (cut up) mix with 3 tsp mayonnaise
   2 slices of rye bread
   ½ cup sliced tomato and lettuce
   1 whole diced mango
   1 cup raspberries

4. (600 calories, 80 gm carb, 35 gm protein, 15 gm fat)

Big Salad:
2 cups mixed greens
½ cup diced carrots
½ cup diced bell peppers
⅓ cup beans
3 oz grilled chicken
4 chopped walnuts
1 diced apple
2 tbsp vinaigrette salad dressing
1 medium nectarine
6-inch whole wheat pita

5. (600 calories, 85 gm carb, 31 gm protein, 15 gm fat)
   3 oz lean roast beef
   2 slices rye bread
   1 tsp mayonnaise
   ½ cup sliced tomato and lettuce
   ½ cup carrot sticks
   1½ cups fresh pineapple
   + 1 cup diced papaya topped with 6 slivered almonds

6. (600 calories, 80 gm carb, 30 gm protein, 15 gm fat)
   3 cups spinach
   1 oz feta cheese
   1 oz firm tofu
   ½ cup water chestnuts

$^1/_2$ cup snap peas
$1^1/_2$ cup mandarin oranges
1 tbsp reduced fat ginger
salad dressing
10 whole grain crackers

7. (600 calories, 80 gm carb,
   31 gm protein, 15 gm fat)

2 slices of whole grain bread
2 oz white meat turkey
1 oz low-fat cheese
2 tsp mayonnaise
$^1/_2$ cup sliced tomato and
lettuce
$1^1/_2$ cups mixed fruit salad
3 whole wheat graham
crackers

## DINNER *(600 calories, approx. 82 gm carbohydrate, 30 gm protein, 16 gm fat):*

1. (600 calories, 85 gm carb,
   28 gm protein, 15 gm fat)
   2 oz cooked chicken (no skin)
   1 cup brown rice
   1 cup green beans sautéed in
   1 tsp olive oil and
   6 slivered almonds
   1 cup mixed greens with
   $^1/_2$ cup chopped tomatoes
   and $^1/_2$ cup chopped
   peppers
   1 tbsp salad dressing
   1 medium apple

2. (600 calories, 85 gm carb, 26
   gm protein, 16 gm fat)
   2 oz lean cooked roast beef
   $^2/_3$ cup brown rice
   $^1/_2$ cup carrots
   $^1/_2$ cup cauliflower
   2 tsp olive oil
   1 whole grain dinner roll
   1 orange

3. (600 calories, 83 gm carb, 29
   gm protein, 16 gm fat)
   2 oz broiled salmon

large sweet potato
1 cup sautéed spinach with 2
tsp olive oil
1 cup sliced tomato
$1^1/_2$ cups diced melon

4. (600 calories, 85 gm carb,
   30 gm protein, 16 gm fat)
   2 oz sautéed shrimp in
   2 tsp olive oil
   $1^1/_2$ cup whole wheat pasta
   $^1/_2$ cup tomato sauce
   $^1/_2$ cup artichoke hearts
   $^1/_2$ cup spinach
   $1^1/_4$ cups sliced strawberries
   1 sliced fresh peach

5. (600 calories, 80 gm carb,
   32 gm protein, 16 gm fat)
   3 oz baked cod
   $^1/_3$ cup cooked whole wheat
   couscous
   2 cups baked winter squash
   1 cup mixed greens (kale,
   collard and mustard) sautéed
   in 3 tsp olive oil
   2 cups cubed papaya

6. (600 calories, 85 gm carb,
   27 gm protein, 16 gm fat)
   2 oz flank steak
   1 cup whole wheat couscous
   2 cups roasted broccoli and
   cauliflower with 2 tsp olive
   oil
   1 1/2 cup raspberries

7. (500 calories, 83 gm carb,
   27 gm protein, 16 gm fat)
   2 oz BBQ chicken
   1 medium corn on the cob
   1 cup baked beans
   1 1/2 cup cucumber and
   tomato salad tossed with
   2 tbsp olive oil–based dressing
   1/2 cup cubed watermelon

**CHOOSE ONE SNACK.**

◆ BETWEEN-MEAL SNACKS *(200 calories, approx. 27 gm carb, 10 gm protein, 6 gm fat)*

1. (200 calories, 27 gm carb, 8 gm protein, 5 gm fat)
   1 cup plain nonfat yogurt
   3/4 cup fresh blackberries
   6 chopped almonds

2. (200 calories, 27 gm carb, 8 gm protein, 5 gm fat)
   1 medium apple
   2 tsp peanut butter
   1 cup skim milk

3. (200 calories, 30 gm carb, 7 gm protein, 7 gm fat)
   1 whole grain English muffin
   1 oz Swiss cheese

4. (200 calories, 27 gm carb, 8 gm protein, 5 gm fat)
   peanut-butter-and-jelly smoothie: Blend 1 cup skim milk +
   1 1/4 cups fresh or frozen strawberries + 2 tsp peanut butter

5. (200 calories, 27 gm carb, 8 gm protein, 5 gm fat)
   6-inch whole wheat pita
   1 sliced apple
   2 tsp peanut butter

6. (200 calories, 27 gm carb, 8 gm protein, 5 gm fat)
   1 slice whole wheat raisin bread topped with 1 sliced kiwi and $1/4$
   cup ricotta cheese

7. (200 calories, 27 gm carb, 8 gm protein, 5 gm fat)
   $1/2$ 6-inch whole wheat pita
   $1/3$ cup humus
   $1/2$ cup carrot sticks

# THREE

# Exercise Prescription for Losing 75 Pounds or More

### ◆ MOST IMPORTANT FACTOR

The most important element as you propel towards your weight loss goals is your *frequency of workouts*. Your ultimate goal is to create an environment that allows you to exercise aerobically, 5 times per week. Depending upon which approach you decide to take with your weight loss plan, simply put, the more you exercise the faster you will shed weight *without* having to severely restrict your food intake.

### ◆ FITNESS EQUIPMENT NEEDED

- Recumbent or upright stationary bike, treadmill, elliptical or cross trainer, or if no access to a piece of aerobic fitness equipment, walk/jog instead.
- Firm exercise mat
- An aerobic bar or one pair of 1-lb dumbbells
- Trampoline (optional)

◆ **PLEASE NOTE:** All of the following exercise regimens can be performed at home, your gym or even while traveling.

## ◆ EXERCISE REGIMEN

- Frequency: 2, 3, 4 or 5 days per week
- Duration: 40 to 60 minutes, depending upon your current level of fitness

***Before starting this or any exercise regimen, get your doctor's approval.***

---

## ◆ WORKOUT #1

Full-Body Routine—2 to 3 days per week, every other day, Mondays, Wednesdays & Fridays or Tuesdays, Thursdays & Saturdays.

1. **Warm-up:** Bike, brisk walk, elliptical or cross trainer for 20 minutes, using low resistance, 70+ RPMs or 3.0+ MPH while walking and 4.5+ MPH if jogging, with no incline.
   - ◆ **PLEASE NOTE:** If you are unable to perform 20 minutes of continuous aerobic exercise, take breaks for a minute or so, catch your breath and resume until you have performed 20 minutes in total.
2. **Stretch:** 4 minutes (see pictures).
3. **Fat Burner:** 5 minutes of biking or other aerobic exercise or bouncing on trampoline—moderate intensity!
4. **Abdominals/Legs:** a) Knees to Elbows—15, rest 30 seconds, repeat 12 reps; b) Crunches: 15, rest 30 seconds, repeat 12 reps.
5. **Legs/Hips:** March in Place—30 to 50 reps. (Bring knees up to at least waist level.)

6. **Fat Burner:** 5 minutes of biking or other aerobic exercise or bouncing on trampoline—moderate intensity!
7. **Upper Body Exercises:** a) Push-outs—25 reps with 1-lb dumbbells or aerobic bar; b) Triceps Kick-backs—25 reps.
8. **Fat Burner:** 5 minutes of biking or other aerobic exercise or bouncing on trampoline—vigorously!
9. **Cool Down:** Bike or walk for 3 minutes, nice and easy.

◆ **IF YOU NEED A BREAK** at any time during your exercise regimen, you can simply get on a stationary bike or any other piece of aerobic equipment or walk 1–3 minutes to allow your heart rate to come down safely before you resume.

And, based upon your current level of fitness, you can either increase or decrease the number of repetitions with each exercise. You should be progressing every two weeks by increasing the speed at which you bike or walk or jog, etc. and increase your repetitions by 1–2 repetitions every 2 weeks eventually trying to get to 50 repetitions for each exercise. Also, if you can only perform a few repetitions of any exercise, don't skip it, do what you can do because as you increase your frequency, the number of repetitions will increase as your fitness level improves.

◆ WORKOUT #2

Aerobic/Abdominals Routine—2 to 3 days per week on days in between Full-Body Routines

1. Bike, brisk walk, elliptical or cross trainer for 30 minutes, moderate intensity.
2. Stretch—4 minutes.
3. Cool Down—3 minutes of easy moving.

### ◆ 1. WARM-UP

### ◆ 2. STRETCH

Stretching takes place after you have warmed up. Hold each stretch for 15–30 seconds. Do not bounce.

---

#### ARM CIRCLES

With arms outstretched, slowly circle your arms backward for 5 revolutions and then 5 revolutions forward.

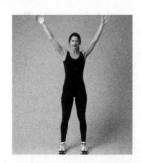

---

#### TRICEPS

With arms overhead, gently pull the right elbow behind your head with your left hand. Hold when you reach a comfortable stretch in the rear shoulder and upper back. Switch arms and repeat.

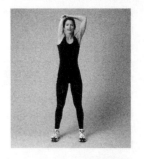

---

#### SHOULDERS, CHEST AND HAMSTRINGS

Grasp hands behind your back, with palms facing each other. Slightly bend your knees and lift arms up as you bend forward at the waist. Hold when you feel a comfortable stretch in the shoulders, chest and hamstrings.

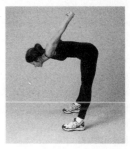

### HAMSTRINGS

In a seated position, with legs straight in front of you, bend forward from the waist and reach towards your toes and hold, without bending knees. You will feel the stretch behind the knees, in the back of the legs, and in the lower back.

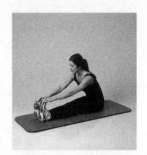

### GROIN

In sitting position, pull your soles of your feet together, and grab hold of your ankles. Gently pull heels toward the groin area. Let your knees relax toward the floor, and gently press your elbows down on your knees to increase the stretch.

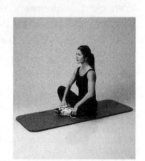

### QUADRICEPS

While lying on your side, pull top leg back by grasping front of your ankle. Gently pull heel toward buttocks. Repeat on other side.

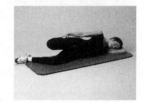

### CALF

With hands and knees on all fours, straighten your body into a V position. With both feet together, bend your left knee and press your right heel towards the ground, stretching your right calf. Repeat on other side.

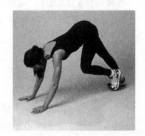

◆ 3. FAT BURNER

◆ 4. ABDOMINALS/LEGS

---

### KNEES-ELBOWS

Lying on floor, with hands clasped at the base of your neck, raise head and shoulder blades off the floor. Raise knees and feet in a tucked position toward elbows, keeping lower back pressed to the floor. Keeping tucked, lower your toes to the ground. Exhale as you raise knees to elbows.

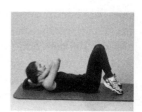
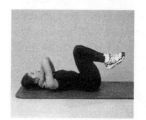

---

### ELBOWS-KNEES (CRUNCHES)

Lying on back, raise knees and feet toward chest in a tucked position. Clasp your hands at the base of your neck. Gently curl your upper body bringing your elbows toward your knees. Slowly lower shoulders to ground. Keep lower half of your body motionless. Exhale as you bring elbows to knees.

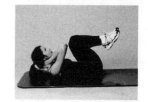
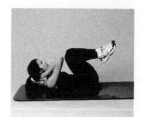

◆ 5. LEGS/HIPS

◆ 6. FAT BURNER

## ◆ 7. UPPER BODY EXERCISES

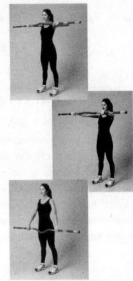

### PUSH-OUTS

Keep your back straight, knees slightly flexed, and feet shoulder width apart.

A. Grip Aerobic Bar, palms facing down, just past shoulder width. Raise bar up just above your chest line with elbows up and wrists firm.

B. Extend arms straight out, holding bar above chest level and exhale.

C. Keeping arms straight, lower bar to front of thighs.

Inhale while you raise arms to first position, exhale as you push out. Keep entire body aligned and still.

### OR

Keep your back straight, knees slightly flexed, and feet shoulder width apart.

A. Grip dumbbells, palms facing down, just past shoulder width. Raise dumbbells up just above your chest line with elbows up and wrists firm.

B. Extend arms straight out, holding dumbbells above chest level and exhale.

C. Keeping arms straight, lower dumbbells to front of thighs.

Inhale while you raise arms to first position, exhale as you push out. Keep entire body aligned and still.

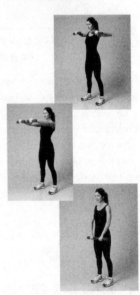

## TRICEP KICKBACKS

Keep back straight, knees flexed, and feet shoulder width apart.

A. Grip Aerobic Bar with arms fully extended at buttocks, palms facing outward.

B. Keeping elbows stationary and wrists firm, raise bar behind your buttocks as far as possible while exhaling. Keeping arms straight, lower bar to buttocks while inhaling.

### OR

Keep back straight, knees flexed, and feet shoulder width apart.

A. Grip dumbbells with arms fully extended at buttocks, palms facing outward.

B. Keeping elbows and wrists firm, raise dumbbells behind your buttocks as far as possible while exhaling. Keeping arms straight, lower dumbbells to buttocks while inhaling.

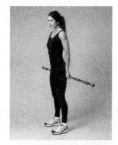

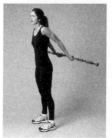

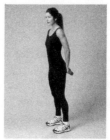

◆ 8. FAT BURNER

◆ 9. COOL DOWN

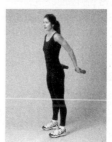

# FOUR

# Diet Plans for Losing 25 to 74 Pounds

## MEAL PLAN TO LOSE 25–74 POUNDS
*RESTRICTIVE APPROACH*

### 1600 CALORIES PER DAY
(221 gm carbohydrate, 80 gm protein, 44 gm fat)

---

**BREAKFAST** *(500 calories, approx. 68 gm carbohydrate, 25 gm protein, 14 gm fat):*

1. (400 calories, 72 gm carb, 24 gm protein, 15 gm fat)
   2¼ cups whole grain cereal (unsweetened, ready-to-eat cereal)
   1 cup skim milk
   1 cup berries
   12 almonds
   1 hard-boiled egg

2. (500 calories, 64 gm carb, 27 gm protein, 12 gm fat)

¾ cup 1% cottage cheese
1 cup berries
1 cup melon
12 almonds
2 slices of whole grain bread

3. (500 calories, 67 gm carb, 26 gm protein, 13 gm fat)
   2 slices of whole grain bread
   1 tbsp peanut butter

1 apple
12 oz low-fat yogurt

4. (500 calories, 65 gm carb,
   28 gm protein, 15 gm fat)
   2 poached eggs
   2 slices of whole grain bread
   3/4 cup plain low-fat yogurt
   1 1/2 cups melon

5. (500 calories, 63 gm carb,
   23 gm protein, 15 gm fat)
   1 1/2 cups cooked oatmeal
   12 chopped walnut halves
   1 chopped red delicious apple
   1/2 cup low-fat cottage cheese

6. (500 calories, 65 gm carb, 25
   gm protein, 10 gm fat)
   Omelet—1 whole egg and
   2 egg whites + 1/2 oz of low-
   fat cheese + 1/2 cup spinach
   + 1/2 cup chopped tomato
   2 slices of whole grain bread
   1 cup sliced strawberries
   1 sliced kiwi

7. (500 calories, 65 gm carb, 22
   gm protein, 16 gm fat)
   2 slices of whole grain bread
   2 oz cheese
   1/2 cup sliced tomato
   2 cups mixed melon

**LUNCH** *(500 calories, approx. 68 gm carbohydrate, 25 gm protein, 14 gm fat):*

1. (500 calories, 65 gm carb,
   22 gm protein, 15 gm fat)
   2 slices of whole grain bread
   2 oz white meat turkey
   1/4 avocado
   1/2 cup sliced tomato and
   lettuce
   1/2 cup unsweetened apple
   sauce with 1/4 cup granola

2. (500 calories, 65 gm carb,
   22 gm protein, 15 gm fat)
   1 whole wheat pita
   2 oz chunk white tuna
   fish
   3 tsp mayonnaise
   1/2 cup mixed shredded
   carrots, lettuce and

celery
24 cherries

3. (500 calories, 65 gm carb,
   22 gm protein, 15 gm fat)
   2 oz of cold chicken (cut up)
   mix with 3 tsp mayonnaise
   2 slices of rye bread
   1/2 cup sliced tomato and
   lettuce
   1 whole diced mango

4. (500 calories, 65 gm carb,
   25 gm protein, 15 gm fat)
   Big Salad:
   2 cups mixed greens
   1/2 cup diced carrots
   1/2 cup diced bell peppers

$^1/_3$ cup beans
2 ounces grilled chicken
4 chopped walnuts
1 diced apple
2 tbsp vinaigrette salad
dressing
1 medium nectarine

5. (500 calories, 70 gm carb,
   24 gm protein, 15 gm fat)
   2 oz lean roast beef
   2 slices rye bread
   1 tsp mayonnaise
   $^1/_2$ cup sliced tomato and
   lettuce
   $^1/_2$ cup carrot sticks
   $1^1/_2$ cup fresh
   pineapple topped
   with 6 slivered
   almonds

6. (500 calories, 60 gm carb,
   28 gm protein, 15 gm fat)
   2 cups spinach
   1 oz feta cheese
   1 oz firm tofu
   $^1/_2$ cup water chestnuts
   $^1/_2$ cup snap peas
   $^3/_4$ cup mandarin oranges
   1 tbsp reduced fat ginger
   salad dressing
   10 whole grain crackers

7. (500 calories, 65 gm carb,
   28 gm protein, 15 gm fat)
   2 slices of whole grain bread
   2 oz white meat turkey
   1 oz low-fat cheese
   2 tsp mayonnaise
   $^1/_2$ cup sliced tomato/lettuce
   $1^1/_2$ cups mixed fruit salad

**DINNER** *(600 calories, approx. 85 gm carbohydrate, 30 gm protein, 16 gm fat):*

1. (600 calories, 85 gm carb,
   28 gm protein, 15 gm fat)
   2 ounces cooked chicken (no skin)
   1 cup brown rice
   1 cup green beans sautéed in
   1 tsp olive oil and
   6 slivered almonds
   1 cup mixed greens with
   $^1/_2$ cup chopped tomatoes
   and $^1/_2$ cup chopped peppers
   1 tbsp salad dressing
   1 medium apple

2. (600 calories, 85 gm carb,
   26 gm protein, 16 gm fat)
   2 oz lean cooked roast beef

   $^2/_3$ cup brown rice
   $^1/_2$ cup carrots
   $^1/_2$ cup cauliflower
   2 tsp olive oil
   1 whole grain dinner roll
   1 orange

3. (600 calories, 83 gm carb,
   29 gm protein, 16 gm fat)
   2 oz broiled salmon
   large sweet potato
   1 cup sautéed spinach with
   2 tsp olive oil
   1 cup sliced tomato
   $1^1/_2$ cups diced melon

4. (600 calories, 85 gm carb,
   30 gm protein, 16 gm fat)
   2 oz sautéed shrimp in
   2 tsp olive oil
   1½ cups whole wheat
   pasta
   ½ cup tomato sauce
   ½ cup artichoke hearts
   ½ cup spinach
   1¼ cups sliced strawberries
   1 sliced fresh peach

5. (600 calories, 80 gm carb,
   32 gm protein, 16 gm fat)
   3 oz baked cod
   ⅓ cup cooked whole wheat
   couscous
   2 cups baked winter squash
   1 cup mixed greens
   (kale, collard and mustard)

sautéed in 3 tsp olive oil
2 cups cubed papaya

6. (600 calories, 85 gm carb,
   27 gm protein, 16 gm fat)
   2 oz flank steak
   1 cup whole wheat couscous
   2 cups roasted broccoli and
   cauliflower with 2 tsp olive oil
   1½ cup raspberries

7. (500 calories 83 gm carb,
   27 gm protein, 16 gm fat)
   2 oz BBQ chicken
   1 medium corn on the cob
   1 cup baked beans
   1½ cups cucumber and
   tomato salad tossed with
   2 tbsp olive oil–based dressing
   ½ cup cubed watermelon

## MEAL PLAN TO LOSE 25–74 POUNDS
*EXCESSIVE APPROACH*

### 2000 CALORIES PER DAY
(274 gm carbohydrate, 98 gm protein, 56 gm fat)

---

**BREAKFAST** *(600 calories, approx. 82 gm carbohydrate,
30 gm protein, 16 gm fat):*

1. (600 calories, 82 gm carb,
   28 gm protein, 15 gm fat)
   2¼ cups whole grain cereal
   (unsweetened, ready-to-eat
   cereal)
   1½ cup skim milk

1¼ cup berries
12 almonds
1 hard-boiled egg

2. (600 calories, 79 gm carb,
   30 gm protein, 17 gm fat)

³/4 cup 1% cottage cheese
1 cup berries
1 cup melon
1 cup Grape-Nuts
12 almonds
2 slices of whole grain bread
2 tsp peanut butter

3. (600 calories, 82 gm carb,
   29 gm protein, 15 gm fat)
   2 slices of whole grain bread
   1 tbsp peanut butter
   1 apple
   12 oz low-fat yogurt
   ¹/2 cup low-fat granola

4. (600 calories, 80 gm carb,
   28 gm protein, 15 gm fat)
   2 poached eggs
   2 slices of whole grain bread
   ³/4 cup plain low-fat yogurt
   1¹/2 cups melon
   1 cup mixed berries

5. (600 calories, 78 gm carb,
   33 gm protein, 15 gm fat)

2 cups cooked oatmeal
12 chopped walnut halves
1 chopped red delicious
apple
³/4 cup low-fat cottage
cheese

6. (600 calories, 80 gm carb,
   27 gm protein, 15 gm fat)
   Omelet—2 whole eggs +
   ¹/2 ounce of low-fat cheese +
   ¹/2 cup spinach + ¹/2 cup
   chopped tomato
   2 slices of whole grain bread
   1 cup sliced strawberries
   1 sliced kiwi
   1 cup cubed melon

7. (600 calories, 84 gm carb,
   30 gm protein, 16 gm fat)
   2 slices of whole grain bread
   2 oz cheese
   ¹/2 cup sliced tomato
   2¹/2 cup mixed melon
   1 cup skim milk

**LUNCH** *(600 calories, approx. 82 gm carbohydrate,
30 gm protein, 16 gm fat):*

1. (600 calories, 80 gm carb,
   29 gm protein, 15 gm fat)
   2 slices of whole grain bread
   3 oz white meat turkey
   ¹/4 avocado
   ¹/2 cup sliced tomato and
   lettuce
   1 cup unsweetened apple
   sauce with ¹/4 cup granola

2. (600 calories, 80 gm carb,
   29 gm protein, 15 gm fat)
   1 whole wheat pita
   3 ounces chunk white tuna
   fish
   3 tsp mayonnaise
   ¹/2 cup mixed shredded
   carrots, lettuce and celery
   36 cherries

3. (600 calories, 80 gm carb,
   29 gm protein, 15 gm fat)
   3 ounces of cold chicken (cut
   up)
   mix with 3 tsp mayonnaise
   2 slices of rye bread
   $1/2$ cup sliced tomato and
   lettuce
   1 whole diced mango
   1 cup raspberries

4. (600 calories, 80 gm carb,
   35 gm protein, 15 gm fat)
   Big Salad:
   2 cups mixed greens
   $1/2$ cup diced carrots
   $1/2$ cup diced bell peppers
   $1/3$ cup beans
   3 oz grilled chicken
   4 chopped walnuts
   1 diced apple
   2 tbsp vinaigrette salad
   dressing
   1 medium nectarine
   6-inch whole wheat pita

5. (600 calories, 85 gm carb,
   31 gm protein, 15 gm fat)
   3 oz lean roast beef
   2 slices rye bread

1 tsp mayonnaise
$1/2$ cup sliced tomato and
lettuce
$1/2$ cup carrot sticks
$1 1/2$ cup fresh pineapple
+ 1 cup diced papaya topped
with 6 slivered almonds

6. (600 calories, 80 gm carb,
   30 gm protein, 15 gm fat)
   3 cups spinach
   1 ounce feta cheese
   1 ounce firm tofu
   $1/2$ cup water chestnuts
   $1/2$ cup snap peas
   $1 1/2$ cup mandarin oranges
   1 tbsp reduced fat ginger
   salad dressing
   10 whole grain crackers

7. (600 calories, 80 gm carb,
   31 gm protein, 15 gm fat)
   2 slices of whole grain bread
   2 oz white meat turkey
   1 oz low-fat cheese
   2 tsp mayonnaise
   $1/2$ cup sliced tomato/lettuce
   $1 1/2$ cups mixed fruit salad
   3 whole wheat graham
   crackers

**DINNER** *(600 calories, approx. 82 gm carbohydrate, 30 gm protein, 16 gm fat):*

1. (600 calories, 85 gm carb, 28
   gm protein, 15 gm fat)
   2 oz cooked chicken (no
   skin)
   1 cup brown rice

1 cup green beans sautéed in
1 tsp olive oil and 6 slivered
almonds
1 cup mixed greens with $1/2$
cup chopped tomatoes and

1/2 cup chopped peppers
1 tbsp salad dressing
1 medium apple

2. (600 calories, 85 gm carb,
   26 gm protein, 16 gm fat)
   2 oz lean cooked roast beef
   2/3 cup brown rice
   1/2 cup carrots
   1/2 cup cauliflower
   2 tsp olive oil
   1 whole grain dinner roll
   1 orange

3. (600 calories 83 gm carb,
   29 gm protein, 16 gm fat)
   2 oz broiled salmon
   large sweet potato
   1 cup sautéed spinach with
   2 tsp olive oil
   1 cup sliced tomato
   1 1/2 cups diced melon

4. (600 calories, 85 gm carb,
   30 gm protein, 16 gm fat)
   2 ounces sautéed shrimp in
   2 tsp olive oil
   1 1/2 cups whole wheat
   pasta
   1/2 cup tomato sauce
   1/2 cup artichoke hearts
   1/2 cup spinach

1 1/4 cups sliced strawberries
1 sliced fresh peach

5. (600 calories, 80 gm carb,
   32 gm protein, 16 gm fat)
   3 oz baked cod
   1/3 cup cooked whole wheat
   couscous
   2 cups baked winter squash
   1 cup mixed greens (kale,
   collard and mustard) sautéed
   in 3 tsp olive oil
   2 cups cubed papaya

6. (600 calories, 85 gm carb,
   27 gm protein, 16 gm fat)
   2 oz flank steak
   1 cup whole wheat couscous
   2 cups roasted broccoli and
   cauliflower with
   2 tsp olive oil
   1 1/2 cup raspberries

7. (500 calories, 83 gm carb,
   27 gm protein, 16 gm fat)
   2 oz BBQ chicken
   1 medium corn on the cob
   1 cup baked beans
   1 1/2 cups cucumber and
   tomato salad tossed with
   2 tbsp olive oil–based dressing
   1/2 cup cubed watermelon

**CHOOSE ONE SNACK FROM PAGES 40–41.**

# MEAL PLAN TO LOSE 25–74 POUNDS
*EQUILIBRIUM APPROACH*

## 1800 CALORIES PER DAY
(247 gm carbohydrate, 90 gm protein, 50 gm fat)

---

**BREAKFAST** *(500 calories, approx. 68 gm carbohydrate, 25 gm protein, 14 gm fat):*

1. (500 calories, 72 gm carb, 24 gm protein, 15 gm fat)
   2$^1$/4 cups whole grain cereal (unsweetened, ready-to-eat cereal)
   1 cup skim milk
   1 cup berries
   12 almonds
   1 hard-boiled egg

2. (500 calories, 64 gm carb, 27 gm protein, 12 gm fat)
   3/4 cup 1% cottage cheese
   1 cup berries
   1 cup melon
   12 almonds
   2 slices of whole grain bread

3. (500 calories, 67 gm carb, 26 gm protein, 13 gm fat)
   2 slices of whole grain bread
   1 tablespoon peanut butter
   1 apple
   12 oz low-fat yogurt

4. (500 calories, 65 gm carb, 28 gm protein, 15 gm fat)
   2 poached eggs
   2 slices of whole grain bread
   3/4 cup plain low-fat yogurt
   1$^1$/2 cups melon

5. (500 calories, 63 gm carb, 23 gm protein, 15 gm fat)
   1$^1$/2 cups cooked oatmeal
   12 chopped walnut halves
   1 chopped red delicious apple
   1/2 cup low-fat cottage cheese

6. (500 calories, 65 gm carb, 25 gm protein, 10 gm fat)
   Omelet—1 whole egg and 2 egg whites +
   1/2 ounce of low-fat cheese +
   1/2 cup spinach +
   1/2 cup chopped tomato
   2 slices of whole grain bread
   1 cup sliced strawberries
   1 sliced kiwi

7. (500 calories, 65 gm carb, 22 gm protein, 16 gm fat)

2 slices of whole grain bread
2 oz cheese

$\frac{1}{2}$ cup sliced tomato
2 cup mixed melon

**LUNCH** *(500 calories, approx. 68 gm carbohydrate, 25 gm protein, 14 gm fat):*

1. (500 calories, 65 gm carb,
   22 gm protein, 15 gm fat)
   2 slices of whole grain bread
   2 oz white meat turkey
   $\frac{1}{4}$ avocado
   $\frac{1}{2}$ cup sliced tomato and
   lettuce
   $\frac{1}{2}$ cup unsweetened apple
   sauce with $\frac{1}{4}$ cup granola

2. (500 calories, 65 gm carb,
   22 gm protein, 15 gm fat)
   1 whole wheat pita
   2 oz chunk white tuna
   fish
   3 tsp mayonnaise
   $\frac{1}{2}$ cup mixed shredded
   carrots, lettuce and
   celery
   24 cherries

3. (500 calories, 65 gm carb,
   22 gm protein, 15 gm fat)
   2 oz of cold chicken
   (cut up)
   mix with 3 tsp mayonnaise
   2 slices of rye bread
   $\frac{1}{2}$ cup sliced tomato and
   lettuce
   1 whole diced mango

4. (500 calories, 65 gm carb,
   25 gm protein, 15 gm fat)

Big Salad:
2 cups mixed greens
$\frac{1}{2}$ cup diced carrots
$\frac{1}{2}$ cup diced bell peppers
$\frac{1}{3}$ cup beans
2 oz grilled chicken
4 chopped walnuts
1 diced apple
2 tbsp vinaigrette salad
dressing
1 medium nectarine

5. (500 calories, 70 gm carb,
   24 gm protein, 15 gm fat)
   2 oz lean roast beef
   2 slices rye bread
   1 tsp mayonnaise
   $\frac{1}{2}$ cup sliced tomato and
   lettuce
   $\frac{1}{2}$ cup carrot sticks
   $1\frac{1}{2}$ cups fresh pineapple
   topped with 6 slivered
   almonds

6. (500 calories, 60 gm carb,
   28 gm protein, 15 gm fat)
   2 cups spinach
   1 oz feta cheese
   1 oz firm tofu
   $\frac{1}{2}$ cup water chestnuts
   $\frac{1}{2}$ cup snap peas
   $\frac{3}{4}$ cup mandarin oranges
   1 tbsp reduced fat ginger

salad dressing
10 whole grain crackers

7. (500 calories, 65 gm carb,
28 gm protein, 15 gm fat)
2 slices of whole grain bread

2 oz white meat turkey
1 oz low-fat cheese
2 tsp mayonnaise
$1/2$ cup sliced tomato and
lettuce
$1 1/2$ cups mixed fruit salad

## DINNER *(600 calories, approx. 85 gm carbohydrate, 30 gm protein, 16 gm fat):*

1. (600 calories 85 gm carb,
28 gm protein, 15 gm fat)
2 oz cooked chicken (no skin)
1 cup brown rice
1 cup green beans sautéed in
1 tsp olive oil and
6 slivered almonds
1 cup mixed greens with
$1/2$ cup chopped tomatoes
and $1/2$ cup chopped peppers
1 tbsp salad dressing
1 medium apple

2. (600 calories 85 gm carb,
26 gm protein, 16 gm fat)
2 ounces lean cooked roast beef
$2/3$ cup brown rice
$1/2$ cup carrots
$1/2$ cup cauliflower
2 tsp olive oil
1 whole grain dinner roll
1 orange

3. (600 calories 83 gm carb,
29 gm protein, 16 gm fat)
2 oz broiled salmon
large sweet potato

1 cup sautéed spinach with
2 tsp olive oil
1 cup sliced tomato
$1 1/2$ cups diced melon

4. (600 calories 85 gm carb,
30 gm protein, 16 gm fat)
2 oz sautéed shrimp in
2 tsp olive oil
$1 1/2$ cup whole wheat pasta
$1/2$ cup tomato sauce
$1/2$ cup artichoke hearts
$1/2$ cup spinach
$1 1/4$ cups sliced strawberries
1 sliced fresh peach

5. (600 calories 80 gm carb,
32 gm protein, 16 gm fat)
3 oz baked cod
$1/3$ cup cooked whole wheat couscous
2 cups baked winter squash
1 cup mixed greens (kale, collard and mustard) sautéed in 3 tsp olive oil
2 cup cubed papaya

6. (600 calories 85 gm carb,
27 gm protein, 16 gm fat)

2 oz flank steak
1 cup whole wheat couscous
2 cups roasted broccoli and
cauliflower with 2 tsp olive oil
1 1/2 cups raspberries

2 oz BBQ chicken
1 medium corn on the cob
1 cup baked beans
1 1/2 cups cucumber and
tomato salad tossed with
2 tbsp olive oil–based
dressing
1/2 cup cubed watermelon

7. (500 calories 83 gm carb,
27 gm protein, 16 gm fat)

**CHOOSE ONE SNACK.**

◆ BETWEEN-MEAL SNACKS *(200 calories, approx. 27 gm carb, 10 gm protein, 6 gm fat)*

1. (200 calories, 27 gm carb, 8 gm protein, 5 gm fat)
   1 cup plain nonfat yogurt
   3/4 cup fresh blackberries
   6 chopped almonds

2. (200 calories, 27 gm carb, 8 gm protein, 5 gm fat)
   1 medium apple
   2 tsp peanut butter
   1 cup skim milk

3. (200 calories, 30 gm carb, 7 gm protein, 7 gm fat)
   1 whole grain English muffin
   1 oz Swiss cheese

4. (200 calories, 27 gm carb, 8 gm protein, 5 gm fat)
   peanut-butter-and-jelly smoothie: Blend 1 cup skim milk +
   1 1/4 cups fresh or frozen strawberries + 2 tsp peanut butter

5. (200 calories, 27 gm carb, 8 gm protein, 5 gm fat)
   6-inch whole wheat pita
   1 sliced apple
   2 tsp peanut butter

6. (200 calories, 27 gm carb, 8 gm protein, 5 gm fat)
   1 slice whole wheat raisin bread topped with 1 sliced kiwi and $\frac{1}{4}$
   cup ricotta cheese

7. (200 calories, 27 gm carb, 8 gm protein, 5 gm fat)
   $\frac{1}{2}$ 6-inch whole wheat pita
   $\frac{1}{3}$ cup humus
   $\frac{1}{2}$ cup carrot sticks

# Exercise Prescription for Losing 25 to 74 Pounds

### ◆ MOST IMPORTANT FACTOR

The most important factors that will insure weight loss for you are two (2) things: First, you need to work out a minimum of 3 days a week performing your full-body routine and second, a decrease in your caloric intake of at least 10%, and both have to be performed simultaneously. Just remember, each day that you don't eat sensibly, you need to counter that with an extra day of working out to insure and maintain long-term weight loss.

### ◆ FITNESS EQUIPMENT NEEDED: (SEE PHOTOS, PAGES 5 & 6)

- Recumbent or upright stationary bike, treadmill, elliptical, crosstrainer or if no access to any equipment, walk/jog instead.
- Firm exercise mat
- Jump rope

- Aerobic bar or 2-lb dumbbells
- Trampoline (optional)

While jumping rope, make sure you jump on a surface that has some give to it such as a wooden floor, short grass, rubberized track or tennis court or the like. DO NOT jump on asphalt or cement. If you don't have access to this type of surface and/or need help in improving your jump rope skills, log onto www.exude.com to view Impact Mat and Jumping Towards Fitness Video.

◆ **PLEASE NOTE:** All of the following exercise regimens can be performed at home, the gym or even while traveling.

### ◆ EXERCISE REGIMEN

- Frequency: 2, 3, 4 or 5 days per week
- Duration: 50 to 60 minutes, depending upon your current level of fitness

***Before starting this or any exercise regimen, get your doctor's approval.***

---

### ◆ WORKOUT # 1

Full-Body Routine—2 to 3 days per week, every other day, Mondays, Wednesdays & Fridays or Tuesdays, Thursdays & Saturdays.

1. **Warm-up:** Bike, brisk walk, light jog, elliptical or cross trainer for 30 minutes with high speed 85+ RPMs, with low resistance, or walk @ 3.5+ MPH or jog @ 5.0+ MPH, with no incline.

♦ **PLEASE NOTE:** If you are unable to perform 30 continuous minutes of aerobic exercise, take a break for a minute or so, then resume until you've completed 30 minutes.

2. **Stretch:** 4 minutes (see pictures).
3. **Fat Burner:** Jump rope or trampoline for 1 minute, then 3 minutes of biking, walking, jogging or aerobic exercise of your choice—with moderate intensity.
4. **Leg/Hips:** a) Standing Knee to Opposite Chest—20–30, b) L-Kicks—20–30, c) March in Place on Toes—50–60.
5. **Upper Body Exercises:** a) Push-outs—35 w/2 lb dumbbells or aerobic bar, b) Front Press—35 reps, c) Upright Rows—35, d) Curls—35, e) Kick-Backs—35.
6. **Fat Burner:** Jump rope or trampoline for 1 minute, then 3 minutes of biking, walking, jogging or aerobic exercise of your choice—with moderate intensity.
7. **Abdominals/Legs:** a) Sit-ups—40–50, b) Leg-outs—20, rest 10 seconds, then repeat 20 reps again, c) V-scissors—20/20, d) Knees to Elbows—20, e) Crunches—20.
8. **Fat Burner:** Jump rope or trampoline for 1 minute, then 3 minutes of biking, walking, jogging or aerobic exercise of your choice—with moderate intensity.
9. **Modified Jumping Jacks:** 40 to 50 reps.
10. **Cool Down:** 3 minutes of biking, or leisurely walking.

♦ **IF YOU NEED A BREAK** at any time during your exercise regimen, you can simply get on a stationary bike or any other piece of aerobic equipment or walk for 1–3 minutes to allow your heart rate to come down safely *before* you resume. Also, if you want to pay more attention to either your upper body, mid-section or lower body, you can perform either more repetitions or do an extra set of exercises that target that region.

Based upon your time allotment and level of fitness, you can either cool down or perform another set of upper body exercises (#5), and another set of abdominals/legs (#7), and then cool down afterwards. If you can perform more repetitions with any exercise, please go ahead and do so. If not, keep track of how many repetitions you do for all of your exercises and as you increase your fitness level you will then be able to comfortably increase the number of repetitions you perform with any and all exercises.

## ◆ WORKOUT # 2

Aerobic/Abdominals/Legs Routine—2 to 3 days per week to be performed on the alternate days and in between Workout #1.

1. Aerobic exercise of your choice for 40 minutes with moderate intensity.
2. Stretch—4 minutes.
3. Modified Jumping Jacks—40 to 50 reps.
4. Abdominals/Legs—Same as #7 in Workout #1.
5. Modified Jumping Jacks—40 to 50 reps.
6. Cool down—3 minutes of leisurely biking or walking.

## ◆ 1. WARM-UP

## ◆ 2. STRETCH

Stretching takes place after you have warmed up. Hold each stretch for 15–30 seconds. Do not bounce.

## ARM CIRCLES

With arms outstretched, slowly circle your arms backward for 5 revolutions and then 5 revolutions forward.

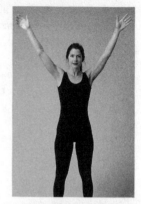

## TRICEPS

With arms overhead, gently pull the right elbow behind your head with your left hand. Hold when you reach a comfortable stretch in the rear shoulder and upper back. Switch arms and repeat.

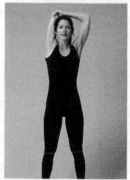

## SHOULDERS, CHEST AND HAMSTRINGS

Grasp hands behind your back, with palms facing each other. Slightly bend your knees and lift arms up as you bend forward at the waist. Hold when you feel a comfortable stretch in the shoulders, chest and hamstrings.

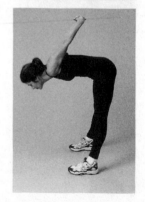

## HAMSTRINGS

In a seated position, with legs straight in front of you, bend forward from the waist and reach towards your toes and hold, without bending knees. You will feel the stretch behind the knees, in the back of the legs, and in the lower back.

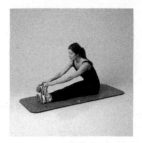

## GROIN

In sitting position, pull your soles of your feet together, and grab hold of your ankles. Gently pull heels toward the groin area. Let your knees relax toward the floor, and gently press your elbows down on your knees to increase the stretch.

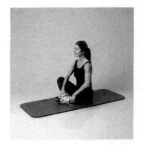

## QUADRICEPS

While lying on your side, pull top leg back by grasping front of your ankle. Gently pull heel toward buttocks. Repeat on other side.

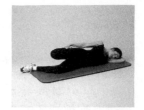

## CALF

With hands and knees on all fours, straighten your body into a V position. With both feet together, bend your left knee and press your right heel towards the ground, stretching your right calf. Repeat on other side.

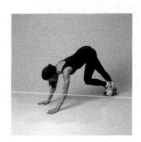

◆ 3. FAT BURNER

◆ 4. LEGS/HIPS

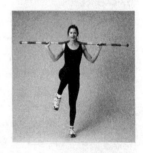

### STANDING KNEE TO OPPOSITE CHEST

Rest the Aerobic Bar on your neck across your shoulders, with feet shoulder width apart.

A. Transfer all weight to your left leg.

B. Raise right knee up toward your left chest to at least waist level.

Lower right foot to starting position, touching the ground while keeping your weight on your left leg throughout the movement. Switch legs and repeat.

### L KICKS

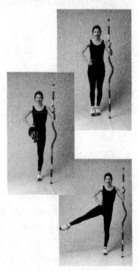

Hold the Aerobic Bar upright with your left hand and place your right hand on your waist.

A. Start with your right leg, point your toe and gently raise your right leg straight as high as possible, without leaning your weight on bar.

B. Then touch to starting position, lightly touching the ground.

C. Pointing your toe, with leg straight, raise the right leg to the side as high as possible, without leaning your weight on bar. Switch legs and repeat.

## PUSH-OUTS

Keep your back straight, knees slightly flexed, and feet shoulder width apart.

A. Grip Aerobic Bar, palms facing down, just past shoulder width. Raise bar up just above your chest line with elbows up and wrists firm.

B. Extend arms straight out, holding bar above chest level and exhale.

C. Keeping arms straight, lower bar to front of thighs.

Inhale while you raise arms to first position, exhale as you push out. Keep entire body aligned and still.

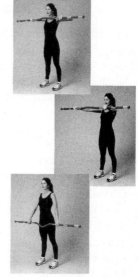

### OR

Keep your back straight, knees slightly flexed, and feet shoulder width apart.

A. Grip dumbbells, palms facing down, just past shoulder width. Raise dumbbells up just above your chest line with elbows up and wrists firm.

B. Extend arms straight out, holding dumbbells above chest level and exhale.

C. Keeping arms straight, lower dumbbells to front of thighs.

Inhale while you raise arms to first position, exhale as you push out. Keep entire body aligned and still.

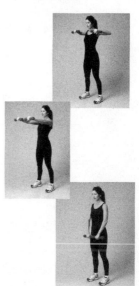

## FRONT PRESS

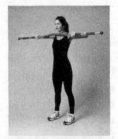

Keep back straight, knees flexed, and feet shoulder width apart.

A. Grip Aerobic Bar just past shoulder width. Rest bar across top of chest.

B. Fully extend arms and raise bar straight up while exhaling. Bend arms and slowly return bar to top of chest while inhaling.

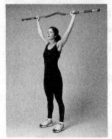

### OR

Keep back straight, knees flexed, and feet shoulder width apart.

A. Grip dumbbells just past shoulder width. Rest dumbbells across top of chest.

B. Fully extend arms and raise dumbbells straight up while exhaling. Bend arms and slowly return dumbbells to top of chest while inhaling.

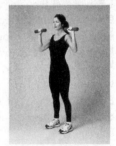

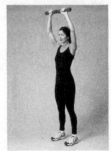

## UPRIGHT ROW

Keep back straight, knees flexed, and feet shoulder width apart.

A. Grip Aerobic Bar, palms facing down, hands six inches apart. Hold bar with arms fully extended at front of thighs.

B. Slowly raise bar up to chin, keeping elbows above bar level while exhaling. Return to starting position while inhaling.

**OR**

Keep back straight, knees flexed, and feet shoulder width apart.

A. Grip dumbbells, palms facing down, hands six inches apart. Hold dumbbells with arms fully extended at front of thighs.

B. Slowly raise dumbbells up to chin, keeping elbows above dumbbell level while exhaling. Return to starting position while inhaling.

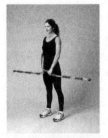

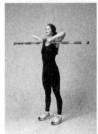

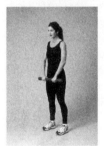

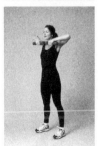

## BICEPS CURL

Keep back straight, knees flexed, and feet shoulder width apart.

A. Grip Aerobic Bar, palms facing up and shoulder width apart. Hold bar with arms fully extended at front of thighs.

B. Keeping elbows stationary and wrists firm, curl bar up to chest while exhaling. Slowly extend arms and return bar to start position while inhaling.

### OR

Keep back straight, knees flexed, and feet shoulder width apart.

A. Grip dumbbells, palms facing up and shoulder width apart. Hold dumbbells with arms fully extended at front of thighs.

B. Keeping elbows stationary and wrists firm, curl dumbbells up to chest while exhaling. Slowly extend arms and return dumbbells to start position while inhaling.

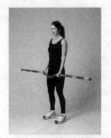

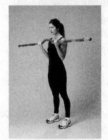

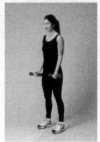

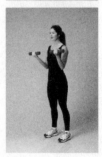

## TRICEP KICKBACKS

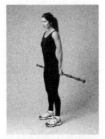

Keep back straight, knees flexed, and feet shoulder width apart.

A. Grip Aerobic Bar with arms fully extended at buttocks, palms facing outward.

B. Keeping elbows stationary and wrists firm, raise bar behind your buttocks as far as possible while exhaling. Keeping arms straight, lower bar to buttocks while inhaling.

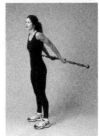

**OR**

Keep back straight, knees flexed, and feet shoulder width apart.

A. Grip dumbbells with arms fully extended at buttocks, palms facing outward.

B. Keeping elbows and wrists firm, raise dumbbells behind your buttocks as far as possible while exhaling. Keeping arms straight, lower dumbbells to buttocks while inhaling.

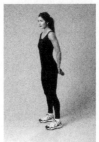

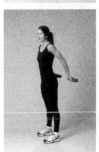

◆ 6. FAT BURNER

◆ 7. ABDOMINAL/LEGS

---

### SIT-UPS

**Beginner:**
Lie on back with knees bent, feet flat on the floor, fingertips on your temples. Slowly raise your head and shoulder blades off the ground. Exhale on the way up and then lower to starting position.

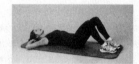
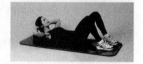

---

**Intermediate:**
Lie on back with knees bent, feet flat on the floor, thumbs clasped with arms extended over your head. Slowly raise your body up, bringing your chest towards your knees. Exhale while sitting up. Slowly lower body to starting position.

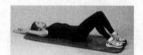
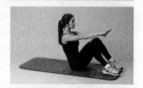

---

**Advanced:**
Lie on back with knees bent, feet flat on the floor, fingertips on your temples, palms facing in. Slowly raise your body up, bringing your chest towards your knees. Exhale while sitting up. Slowly lower body to starting position.

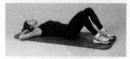
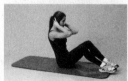

## LEG-OUTS

Lying on your back, with hands under buttocks, palms down, bring both knees in toward your chest. Slowly straighten legs out with toes pointed. Inhale while bringing knees toward chest, exhale as you straighten legs. Beginner should straighten legs out at a higher angle. As you get stronger, try to bring legs lower to the ground.

*Beginners*

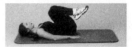

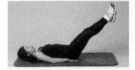

*Intermediate*

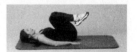

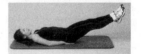

*Advanced*

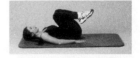

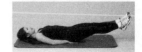

## V-SCISSORS

Lying on your back, hands at your side. Raise your legs to a 90 degree angle. While keeping back on floor, toes pointed, slowly open legs as wide apart as possible. Bring legs back together keeping toes pointed while exhaling.

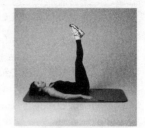

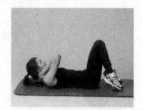

## KNEES-ELBOWS

Lying on floor, with hands clasped at the base of your neck, raise head and shoulder blades off the floor. Raise knees and feet in a tucked position toward elbows, keeping lower back pressed to the floor. Keeping tucked, lower your toes to the ground. Exhale as you raise knees to elbows.

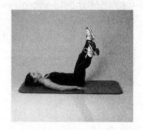

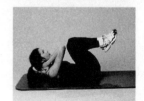

## ELBOWS-KNEES (CRUNCHES)

Lying on back, raise knees and feet toward chest in a tucked position. Clasp your hands at the base of your neck. Gently curl your upper body bringing your elbows toward your knees. Slowly lower shoulders to ground. Keep lower half of your body motionless. Exhale as you bring elbows to knees.

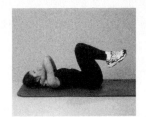

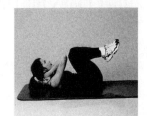

◆ 8. FAT BURNER

◆ 9. MODIFIED JUMPING JACKS

## JUMPING JACKS

A. Stand with back straight, knees slightly flexed, feet wider than shoulder width apart, and arms fully extended over head.
B. Jump one inch off ground while bringing legs together and lowering arms straight to your sides.
C. Jump one inch off ground and return to starting position.

◆ 10. COOL DOWN

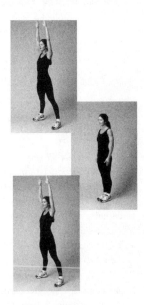

# SIX

# Diet Plans for Losing Less Than 25 Pounds

## MEAL PLAN TO LOSE LESS THAN 25 POUNDS
### *RESTRICTIVE APPROACH*

### 1400 CALORIES PER DAY
(221 gm carbohydrate, 80 gm protein, 44 gm fat)

---

**BREAKFAST** *(400 calories, approx. 55 gm carbohydrate, 20 gm protein, 11 gm fat):*

1. (400 calories, 57 gm carb, 14 gm protein, 10 gm fat)
   1$^1$/2 cups whole grain cereal (unsweetened, ready-to-eat cereal)
   1 cup skim milk
   1 cup berries
   12 almonds

2. (400 calories, 45 gm carb, 20 gm protein, 12 gm fat)
   $^1$/2 cup 1% cottage cheese
   1 cup berries
   12 almonds
   2 slices of whole grain bread

3. (400 calories, 55 gm carb, 18 gm protein, 8 gm fat)
   2 slices of whole grain bread
   1 tbs peanut butter
   1 apple
   6 oz low-fat yogurt

4. (400 calories, 53 gm carb,
   20 gm protein, 10 gm fat)
   2 poached eggs
   2 slices of whole grain bread
   1 1/2 cups melon

5. (400 calories, 48 gm carb,
   20 gm protein, 11 gm fat)
   1 cup cooked oatmeal
   9 chopped walnut halves
   1 chopped red delicious
   apple
   1/2 cup low-fat cottage
   cheese

6. (400 calories, 45 gm carb,
   23 gm protein, 10 gm fat)
   Omelet—1 whole egg and
   2 egg whites + 1/2 oz of low-
   fat cheese + 1/2 cup spinach
   2 slices of whole grain bread
   1 cup sliced strawberries

7. (400 calories, 50 gm carb,
   19 gm protein, 11 gm fat)
   2 slices of whole grain bread
   1 1/2 oz cheese
   1/2 cup sliced tomato
   1 cup mixed melon

**LUNCH** *(500 calories, approx. 68 gm carbohydrate, 25 gm
protein, 14 gm fat):*

1. (500 calories, 65 gm carb,
   22 gm protein, 15 gm fat)
   2 slices of whole grain bread
   2 oz white meat turkey
   1/4 avocado
   1/2 cup sliced tomato and
   lettuce
   1/2 cup unsweetened apple
   sauce with 1/4 cup granola

2. (500 calories, 65 gm carb,
   22 gm protein, 15 gm fat)
   1 whole wheat pita
   2 oz chunk white tuna fish
   3 tsp mayonnaise
   1/2 cup mixed shredded
   carrots, lettuce and celery
   24 cherries

3. (500 calories, 65 gm carb,
   22 gm protein, 15 gm fat)

   2 oz of cold chicken (cut up)
   mix with 3 tsp mayonnaise
   2 slices of rye bread
   1/2 cup sliced tomato and
   lettuce
   1 whole diced mango

4. (500 calories, 65 gm carb,
   25 gm protein, 15 gm fat)
   Big Salad:
   2 cups mixed greens
   1/2 cup diced carrots
   1/2 cup diced bell
   peppers
   1/3 cup beans
   2 oz grilled chicken
   4 chopped walnuts
   1 diced apple
   2 tbsp vinaigrette salad
   dressing
   1 medium nectarine

5. (500 calories, 70 gm carb,
   24 gm protein, 15 gm fat)
   2 oz lean roast beef
   2 slices rye bread
   1 tsp mayonnaise
   $1/2$ cup sliced tomato and
   lettuce
   $1/2$ cup carrot sticks
   $1^1/2$ cup fresh pineapple
   topped with 6 slivered
   almonds

6. (500 calories, 60 gm carb,
   28 gm protein, 15 gm fat)
   2 cups spinach
   1 ounce feta cheese
   1 ounce firm tofu

$1/2$ cup water chestnuts
$1/2$ cup snap peas
$3/4$ cup mandarin oranges
1 tbsp reduced fat ginger
salad dressing
10 whole grain crackers

7. (500 calories, 65 gm carb,
   28 gm protein, 15 gm fat)
   2 slices of whole grain bread
   2 oz white meat turkey
   1 oz low-fat cheese
   2 tsp mayonnaise
   $1/2$ cup sliced tomato and
   lettuce
   $1^1/2$ cups mixed fruit salad

**DINNER** (*500 calories, approx. 68 gm carbohydrate, 25 gm protein, 14 gm fat*):

1. (500 calories 65 gm carb,
   26 gm protein, 15 gm fat)
   2 oz cooked chicken (no skin)
   $2/3$ cup brown rice
   $1/2$ cup green beans sautéed
   in 1 tsp olive oil and 6
   slivered almonds
   1 cup mixed greens with
   $1/2$ cup chopped tomatoes
   and $1/2$ cup chopped peppers
   1 tbsp salad dressing
   1 medium apple

2. (500 calories, 70 gm carb,
   23 gm protein, 14 gm fat)
   2 oz lean cooked roast beef
   $1/3$ cup brown rice
   $1/2$ cup carrots

$1/2$ cup cauliflower
$1^1/2$ tsp olive oil
1 whole grain dinner roll
1 orange

3. (500 calories 68 gm carb,
   29 gm protein, 14 gm fat)
   2 oz broiled salmon
   large sweet potato
   1 cup sautéed spinach with
   $1^1/2$ tsp olive oil
   1 cup sliced tomato
   $1/2$ cup diced melon

4. (500 calories, 50 gm carb,
   25 gm protein, 14 gm fat)
   2 oz sautéed shrimp in
   $1^1/2$ tsp olive oil

1 cup whole wheat pasta
1/2 cup tomato sauce
1/2 cup artichoke hearts
1 1/4 cups sliced strawberries

5. (500 calories, 65 gm carb,
   29 gm protein, 14 gm fat)
   3 oz baked cod
   2 cups baked winter squash
   1 cup mixed greens (kale,
   collard mustard) sautéed in
   2 1/2 tsp olive oil
   2 cup cubed papaya

6. (500 calories, 70 gm carb,
   27 gm protein, 14 gm fat)

2 oz flank steak
1 cup whole wheat couscous
2 cups roasted broccoli and
cauliflower with
1 1/2 tsp olive oil
3/4 cup raspberries

7. (500 calories 68 gm carb,
   27 gm protein, 14 gm fat)
   2 oz BBQ chicken
   1 medium corn on the cob
   2/3 cup baked beans
   1 1/2 cups cucumber and
   tomato salad tossed with 1 1/2
   tbsp olive oil–based dressing
   1/2 cup cubed watermelon

# MEAL PLAN TO LOSE LESS THAN 25 POUNDS
*EXCESSIVE APPROACH*

## 1800 CALORIES PER DAY
(247 gm carbohydrate, 90 gm protein, 50 gm fat)

---

**BREAKFAST** *(500 calories, approx. 68 gm carbohydrate, 25 gm protein, 14 gm fat):*

1. (500 calories, 72 gm carb,
   24 gm protein, 15 gm fat)
   2 1/4 cups whole grain cereal
   (unsweetened, ready-to-eat
   cereal)
   1 cup skim milk
   1 cup berries
   12 almonds
   1 hard-boiled egg

2. (500 calories, 64 gm carb,
   27 gm protein, 12 gm fat)
   3/4 cup 1% cottage cheese
   1 cup berries
   1 cup melon
   12 almonds
   2 slices of whole grain bread

3. (500 calories, 67 gm carb,
   26 gm protein, 13 gm fat)

2 slices of whole grain bread
1 tbs peanut butter
1 apple
12 oz low-fat yogurt

4. (500 calories, 65 gm carb,
   28 gm protein, 15 gm fat)
   2 poached eggs
   2 slices of whole grain bread
   3/4 cup plain low-fat yogurt
   1 1/2 cups melon

5. (500 calories, 63 gm carb,
   23 gm protein, 15 gm fat)
   1 1/2 cups cooked oatmeal
   12 chopped walnut halves
   1 chopped red delicious
   apple
   1/2 cup low-fat cottage cheese

6. (500 calories, 65 gm carb,
   25 gm protein, 10 gm fat)
   Omelet—1 whole egg and
   2 egg whites +
   1/2 ounce of low-fat cheese +
   1/2 cup spinach +
   1/2 cup chopped tomato
   2 slices of whole grain bread
   1 cup sliced strawberries
   1 sliced kiwi

7. (500 calories, 65 gm carb,
   22 gm protein, 16 gm fat)
   2 slices of whole grain bread
   2 oz cheese
   1/2 cup sliced tomato
   2 cups mixed melon

## LUNCH *(500 calories, approx. 68 gm carbohydrate, 25 gm protein, 14 gm fat):*

1. (500 calories, 65 gm carb,
   22 gm protein, 15 gm fat)
   2 slices of whole grain bread
   2 oz white meat turkey
   1/4 avocado
   1/2 cup sliced tomato and
   lettuce
   1/2 cup unsweetened apple
   sauce with 1/4 cup granola

2. (500 calories, 65 gm carb,
   22 gm protein, 15 gm fat)
   1 whole wheat pita
   2 oz chunk white tuna fish
   3 tsp mayonnaise
   1/2 cup mixed shredded

carrots, lettuce and celery
24 cherries

3. (500 calories, 65 gm carb,
   22 gm protein, 15 gm fat)
   2 ounces of cold chicken
   (cut up)
   mix with 3 tsp mayonnaise
   2 slices of rye bread
   1/2 cup sliced tomato and
   lettuce
   1 whole diced mango

4. (500 calories, 65 gm carb,
   25 gm protein, 15 gm fat)
   Big Salad:

2 cups mixed greens
$1/2$ cup diced carrots
$1/2$ cup diced bell peppers
$1/3$ cup beans
2 oz grilled chicken
4 chopped walnuts
1 diced apple
2 tbsp vinaigrette salad dressing
1 medium nectarine

5. (500 calories, 70 gm carb,
   24 gm protein, 15 gm fat)
   2 oz lean roast beef
   2 slices rye bread
   1 tsp mayonnaise
   $1/2$ cup sliced tomato and
   lettuce
   $1/2$ cup carrot sticks
   $1 1/2$ cup fresh pineapple
   topped with 6 slivered
   almonds

6. (500 calories, 60 gm carb,
   28 gm protein, 15 gm fat)
   2 cups spinach
   1 oz feta cheese
   1 oz firm tofu
   $1/2$ cup water chestnuts
   $1/2$ cup snap peas
   $3/4$ cup mandarin oranges
   1 tbsp reduced fat ginger
   salad dressing
   10 whole grain crackers

7. (500 calories, 65 gm carb,
   28 gm protein, 15 gm fat)
   2 slices of whole grain bread
   2 oz white meat turkey
   1 oz low-fat cheese
   2 tsp mayonnaise
   $1/2$ cup sliced tomato and
   lettuce
   $1 1/2$ cups mixed fruit salad

**DINNER** *(600 calories, approx. 85 gm carbohydrate, 30 gm protein, 16 gm fat):*

1. (600 calories, 85 gm carb,
   28 gm protein, 15 gm fat)
   2 ounces cooked chicken
   (no skin)
   1 cup brown rice
   1 cup green beans sautéed in
   1 tsp olive oil and
   6 slivered almonds
   1 cup mixed greens with
   $1/2$ cup chopped tomatoes
   and $1/2$ cup chopped
   peppers
   1 tbsp salad dressing
   1 medium apple

2. (600 calories, 85 gm carb,
   26 gm protein, 16 gm fat)
   2 oz lean cooked roast beef
   $2/3$ cup brown rice
   $1/2$ cup carrots
   $1/2$ cup cauliflower
   2 tsp olive oil
   1 whole grain dinner roll
   1 orange

3. (600 calories, 83 gm carb,
   29 gm protein, 16 gm fat)
   2 oz broiled salmon
   large sweet potato

1 cup sautéed spinach with
2 tsp olive oil
1 cup sliced tomato
1 1/2 cups diced melon

1 cup mixed greens
(kale, collard and mustard)
sautéed in 3 tsp olive oil
2 cups cubed papaya

4. (600 calories, 85 gm carb,
   30 gm protein, 16 gm fat)
   2 oz sautéed shrimp in
   2 tsp olive oil
   1 1/2 cup whole wheat pasta
   1/2 cup tomato sauce
   1/2 cup artichoke hearts
   1/2 cup spinach
   1 1/4 cups sliced
   strawberries
   1 sliced fresh peach

6. (600 calories 85 gm carb,
   27 gm protein, 16 gm fat)
   2 oz flank steak
   1 cup whole wheat couscous
   2 cups roasted broccoli
   and cauliflower with
   2 tsp olive oil
   1 1/2 cups raspberries

7. (500 calories 83 gm carb,
   27 gm protein, 16 gm fat)
   2 oz BBQ chicken
   1 medium corn on the cob
   1 cup baked beans
   1 1/2 cups cucumber and
   tomato salad tossed with 2
   tbsp olive oil–based dressing
   1/2 cup cubed watermelon

5. (600 calories, 85 gm carb,
   32 gm protein, 16 gm fat)
   3 oz baked cod
   1/3 cup cooked whole wheat
   couscous
   2 cups baked winter squash

**CHOOSE ONE SNACK FROM PAGES 67–68.**

## MEAL PLAN TO LOSE LESS THAN 25 POUNDS
*EQUILIBRIUM APPROACH*

### 1600 CALORIES PER DAY
(221 gm carbohydrate, 80 gm protein, 44 gm fat)

---

**BREAKFAST** *(400 calories, approx. 55 gm carbohydrate, 20 gm protein, 11 gm fat):*

1. (400 calories, 57 gm carb,
   14 gm protein, 10 gm fat)
   1 1/2 cups whole grain cereal

   (unsweetened, ready-to-eat
   cereal)
   1 cup skim milk

1 cup berries
12 almonds

2. (400 calories, 45 gm carb,
   20 gm protein, 12 gm fat)
   ½ cup 1% cottage cheese
   1 cup berries
   12 almonds
   2 slices of whole grain
   bread

3. (400 calories, 55 gm carb,
   18 gm protein, 8 gm fat)
   2 slices of whole grain
   bread
   1 tbsp peanut butter
   1 apple
   6 oz low-fat yogurt

4. (400 calories, 53 gm carb,
   20 gm protein, 10 gm fat)
   2 poached eggs
   2 slices of whole grain bread
   1½ cups melon

5. (400 calories, 48 gm carb,
   20 gm protein, 11 gm fat)
   1 cup cooked oatmeal
   9 chopped walnut halves
   1 chopped red delicious
   apple
   ½ cup low-fat cottage
   cheese

6. (400 calories, 45 gm carb,
   23 gm protein, 10 gm fat)
   Omelet—1 whole egg and
   2 egg whites +
   ½ ounce of low-fat cheese +
   ½ cup spinach
   2 slices of whole grain bread
   1 cup sliced strawberries

7. (400 calories, 50 gm carb,
   19 gm protein, gm fat)
   2 slices of whole grain bread
   1½ oz cheese
   ½ cup sliced tomato
   1 cup mixed melon

**LUNCH** *(500 calories, approx. 68 gm carbohydrate, 25 gm protein, 14 gm fat):*

1. (500 calories, 65 gm carb,
   22 gm protein, 15 gm fat)
   2 slices of whole grain
   bread
   2 oz white meat turkey
   ¼ avocado
   ½ cup sliced tomato and
   lettuce
   ½ cup unsweetened
   apple sauce with
   ¼ cup granola

2. (500 calories, 65 gm carb,
   22 gm protein, 15 gm fat)
   1 whole wheat pita
   2 oz chunk white tuna fish
   3 tsp mayonnaise
   ½ cup mixed shredded
   carrots, lettuce and celery
   24 cherries

3. (500 calories, 65 gm carb,
   22 gm protein, 15 gm fat)

2 oz of cold chicken (cut up)
mix with 3 tsp mayonnaise
2 slices of rye bread
1/2 cup sliced tomato and
lettuce
1 whole diced mango

4. (500 calories, 65 gm carb,
   25 gm protein, 15 gm fat)
   Big Salad:
   2 cups mixed greens
   1/2 cup diced carrots
   1/2 cup diced bell peppers
   1/3 cup beans
   2 oz grilled chicken
   4 chopped walnuts
   1 diced apple
   2 tbsp vinaigrette salad dressing
   1 medium nectarine

5. (500 calories, 70 gm carb,
   24 gm protein, 15 gm fat)
   2 oz lean roast beef
   2 slices of rye bread
   1 tsp mayonnaise
   1/2 cup sliced tomato and
   lettuce

1/2 cup carrot sticks
1 1/2 cup fresh pineapple
topped with 6 slivered
almonds

6. (500 calories, 60 gm carb,
   28 gm protein, 15 gm fat)
   2 cups spinach
   1 oz feta cheese
   1 oz firm tofu
   1/2 cup water chestnuts
   1/2 cup snap peas
   3/4 cup mandarin oranges
   1 tbsp reduced fat ginger
   salad dressing
   10 whole grain crackers

7. (500 calories, 65 gm carb,
   28 gm protein, 15 gm fat)
   2 slices of whole grain
   bread
   2 oz white meat turkey
   1 oz low-fat cheese
   2 tsp mayonnaise
   1/2 cup sliced tomato and
   lettuce
   1 1/2 cups mixed fruit salad

**DINNER** (*500 calories, approx. 68 gm carbohydrate, 25 gm
protein, 14 gm fat*):

1. (500 calories, 65 gm carb,
   26 gm protein, 15 gm fat)
   2 oz cooked chicken (no skin)
   2/3 cup brown rice
   1/2 cup green beans sautéed
   in 1 tsp olive oil and
   6 slivered almonds
   1 cup mixed greens with

1/2 cup chopped tomatoes
and 1/2 cup chopped peppers
1 tbsp salad dressing
1 medium apple

2. (500 calories, 70 gm carb,
   23 gm protein, 14 gm fat)
   2 oz lean cooked roast beef

$^1/_3$ cup brown rice
$^1/_2$ cup carrots
$^1/_2$ cup cauliflower
$1^1/_2$ tsp olive oil
1 whole grain dinner roll
1 orange

3. (500 calories, 68 gm carb,
   29 gm protein, 14 gm fat)
   2 oz broiled salmon
   large sweet potato
   1 cup sautéed spinach with
   $1^1/_2$ tsp olive oil
   1 cup sliced tomato
   $^1/_2$ cup diced melon

4. (500 calories, 50 gm carb,
   25 gm protein, 14 gm fat)
   2 oz sautéed shrimp in
   $1^1/_2$ tsp olive oil
   1 cup whole wheat pasta
   $^1/_2$ cup tomato sauce
   $^1/_2$ cup artichoke hearts
   $1^1/_4$ cups sliced strawberries

5. (500 calories, 65 gm carb,
   29 gm protein, 14 gm fat)

3 oz baked cod
2 cups baked winter squash
1 cup mixed greens
(kale, collard mustard)
sautéed in $2^1/_2$ tsp olive oil
2 cups cubed papaya

6. (500 calories, 70 gm carb,
   27 gm protein, 14 gm fat)
   2 oz flank steak
   1 cup whole wheat couscous
   2 cups roasted broccoli
   and cauliflower with
   $1^1/_2$ tsp olive oil
   $^3/_4$ cup raspberries

7. (500 calories, 68 gm carb,
   27 gm protein, 14 gm fat)
   2 oz BBQ chicken
   1 medium corn on the
   cob
   $^2/_3$ cup baked beans
   $1^1/_2$ cup cucumber and
   tomato salad tossed with $1^1/_2$
   tbsp olive oil–based dressing
   $^1/_2$ cup cubed
   watermelon

**CHOOSE ONE SNACK.**

◆ BETWEEN-MEAL SNACKS *(200 calories, approx. 27 gm carb, 10 gm protein, 6 gm fat)*

1. (200 calories, 27 gm carb, 8 gm protein, 5 gm fat)
   1 cup plain nonfat yogurt
   $^3/_4$ cup fresh blackberries
   6 chopped almonds

2. (200 calories, 27 gm carb, 8 gm protein, 5 gm fat)
   1 medium apple
   2 tsp peanut butter
   1 cup skim milk

3. (200 calories, 30 gm carb, 7 gm protein, 7 gm fat)
   1 whole grain English muffin
   1 oz Swiss cheese

4. (200 calories, 27 gm carb, 8 gm protein, 5 gm fat)
   peanut-butter-and-jelly smoothie: Blend 1 cup skim milk +
   $1\frac{1}{4}$ cups fresh or frozen strawberries + 2 tsp peanut butter

5. (200 calories, 27 gm carb, 8 gm protein, 5 gm fat)
   6-inch whole wheat pita
   1 sliced apple
   2 tsp peanut butter

6. (200 calories, 27 gm carb, 8 gm protein, 5 gm fat)
   1 slice whole wheat raisin bread topped with 1 sliced kiwi and $\frac{1}{4}$
   cup ricotta cheese

7. (200 calories, 27 gm carb, 8 gm protein, 5 gm fat)
   $\frac{1}{2}$ 6-inch whole wheat pita
   $\frac{1}{3}$ cup humus
   $\frac{1}{2}$ cup carrot sticks

# Exercise Prescription for Losing Less Than 25 Pounds

### ◆ MOST IMPORTANT FACTOR

As you get nearer your goal of your "ideal weight," your caloric intake becomes just as important as your exercise frequency. But the most important factor for you to focus on with regard to your exercise regimen aside from being consistent is the *intensity* at which you work out. The more intense your exercise, the more calories you will burn in the same amount of time. As you become more fit, you must also increase your effort to insure that you are creating a deficit of calories for that same time period.

### ◆ FITNESS EQUIPMENT NEEDED

- Recumbent or upright stationary bike, treadmill, elliptical, crosstrainer or if no access to a piece of aerobic fitness equipment, walk/jog instead.
- Firm exercise mat
- Aerobic bar or one pair of 3-lb dumbbells
- Jump rope

While jumping rope, make sure you are doing so on a surface that has a give to it such as a wooden floor, short grass, rubberized track or tennis court or the like. DO NOT jump rope on asphalt or cement. If you don't have access to this type of surface and/or need help in improving your jump rope skills, log onto www.exude.com to view Impact Mat and Jumping Towards Fitness Video.

◆ **PLEASE NOTE:** All of the following exercise regimens can be performed at home, your gym or even while traveling.

◆ EXERCISE REGIMEN

- Frequency: 2, 3, 4 or 5 days per week
- Duration: 60 minutes

***Before starting this or any exercise program, get your doctor's approval.***

---

◆ WORKOUT #1

Full-body Routine—2–3 days per week, every other day, Mondays, Wednesdays & Fridays or Tuesdays, Thursdays & Saturdays.

1. **Warm-up:** Bike, jog, brisk walk, elliptical or cross trainer for 25 minutes, using low-moderate resistance, 90+ RPMs or 4.0 MPH while walking and 5.5+ MPH if jogging with no incline.
2. **Stretch:** 3 minutes (see pictures).
3. **Fat Burner:** Jump rope for 3 minutes or bike or any other aerobic activity of your choice for 4 minutes— vigorously!
4. **Upper Body Exercises:** a) Push-outs—40–50 reps with aerobic bar or 3-lb dumbbells, b) Behind Neck Press—40–50 reps, c) Front Press—40–50 reps, d) Upright Rows—40–50 reps, e) Curls—40–50 reps, f) Kick-backs—30 reps.

5. **Jumping Jacks:** 60–75 reps.
6. **Fat Burner:** Jump rope for 3 minutes or bike or any other aerobic activity of your choice for 4 minutes—vigorously!
7. **Legs/Hips:** a) Standing Knee to Opposite Chest 40 reps, b) L-kicks—40, c) March in Place on Toes—75.
8. **Abdominals/Legs:** a) Sit-ups—50, b) Leg-outs—40–50, c) Vertical Scissors—30–40, d) Elbows to Knees—30, e) Knees to Elbows—30, f) Repeat Sit-ups—25.
9. **Fat Burner:** Jump rope for 5–10 minutes or bike or any other aerobic activity of your choice for 10 minutes—vigorously!
10. **Cool Down**—Easy biking, walking or the like for 3 mins.

◆ **IF YOU NEED A BREAK** at any time during your exercise regimen, you can simply get on a stationary bike or any other piece of aerobic equipment or walk for 1–3 minutes to allow your heart rate to come down safely before you resume. Also, if you want to pay more attention to either your upper body, mid-section or lower body, you can perform either more repetitions or do an extra set of exercises that target that region.

Based on your time allotment and level of fitness, you can either cool down or perform another upper body routine (#4), and another set of Abdominals/Legs (#8), and then cool down.

◆ WORKOUT #2

Aerobic Routine—2 to 3 days per week to be performed on the alternate days and in between Workout #1.

1. Aerobic exercise of your choice for 50 minutes.
2. Stretch—3 minutes.
3. March in place—75–100 reps.
4. Jumping jacks—75–100.
5. Cool down—nice and easy for 3 minutes of biking, walking or the like.

◆ 1. WARM-UP

◆ 2. STRETCHES *(Follow instructions on page 46 for arm circles, triceps and shoulders, chest and hamstring stretches.)*

### HAMSTRINGS

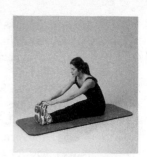

In a seated position, with legs straight in front of you, bend forward from the waist and reach towards your toes and hold, without bending knees. You will feel the stretch behind the knees, in the back of the legs, and in the lower back.

### GROIN

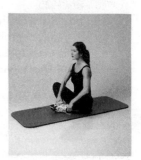

In sitting position, pull your soles of your feet together, and grab hold of your ankles. Gently pull heels toward the groin area. Let your knees relax toward the floor, and gently press your elbows down on your knees to increase the stretch.

### QUADRICEPS

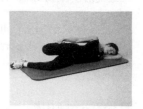

While lying on your side, pull top leg back by grasping front of your ankle. Gently pull heel toward buttocks. Repeat on other side.

### CALF

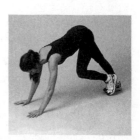

With hands and knees on all fours, straighten your body into a V position. With both feet together, bend your left knee and press your right heel towards the ground, stretching your right calf. Repeat on other side.

### ◆ 3. FAT BURNER

### ◆ 4. UPPER BODY EXERCISES

---

#### PUSH-OUTS

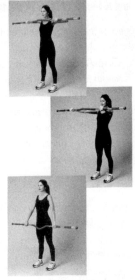

Keep your back straight, knees slightly flexed, and feet shoulder width apart.

A. Grip Aerobic Bar, palms facing down, just past shoulder width. Raise bar up just above your chest line with elbows up and wrists firm.

B. Extend arms straight out, holding bar above chest level and exhale.

C. Keeping arms straight, lower bar to front of thighs.

Inhale while you raise arms to first position, exhale as you push out. Keep entire body aligned and still.

#### OR

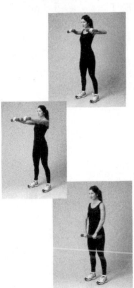

Keep your back straight, knees slightly flexed, and feet shoulder width apart.

A. Grip dumbbells, palms facing down, just past shoulder width. Raise dumbbells up just above your chest line with elbows up and wrists firm.

B. Extend arms straight out, holding dumbbells above chest level and exhale.

C. Keeping arms straight, lower dumbbells to front of thighs.

Inhale while you raise arms to first position, exhale as you push out. Keep entire body aligned and still.

## BEHIND THE NECK PRESS

Keep back straight, knees flexed, and feet shoulder width apart.

A. Grip Aerobic Bar just past shoulder width and place behind neck and shoulders.

B. Fully extend arms and raise bar straight up behind head, while exhaling. Bend arms and slowly return bar to behind neck while inhaling.

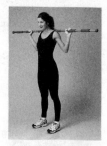

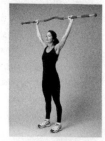

### OR

Keep back straight, knees flexed, and feet shoulder width apart.

A. Grip dumbbells just past shoulder width and place behind neck and shoulders.

B. Fully extend arms and raise dumbbells straight up behind head, while exhaling. Bend arms and slowly return dumbbells to behind neck while inhaling.

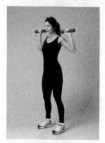

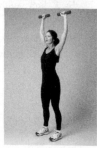

## FRONT PRESS

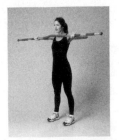

Keep back straight, knees flexed, and feet shoulder width apart.

A. Grip Aerobic Bar just past shoulder width. Rest bar across top of chest.

B. Fully extend arms and raise bar straight up while exhaling. Bend arms and slowly return bar to top of chest while inhaling.

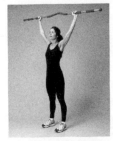

### OR

Keep back straight, knees flexed, and feet shoulder width apart.

A. Grip dumbbells just past shoulder width. Rest dumbbells across top of chest.

B. Fully extend arms and raise dumbbells straight up behind head, while exhaling. Bend arms and slowly return dumbbells to top of chest while inhaling.

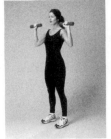

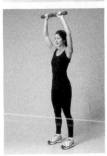

## UPRIGHT ROW

Keep back straight, knees flexed, and feet shoulder width apart.

A. Grip Aerobic Bar, palms facing down, hands six inches apart. Hold bar with arms fully extended at front of thighs.

B. Slowly raise bar up to chin, keeping elbows above bar level while exhaling. Return to starting position while inhaling.

**OR**

Keep back straight, knees flexed, and feet shoulder width apart.

A. Grip dumbbells, palms facing down, hands six inches apart. Hold dumbbells with arms fully extended at front of thighs.

B. Slowly raise dumbbells up to chin, keeping elbows above dumbbell level while exhaling. Return to starting position while inhaling.

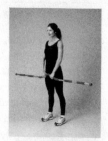
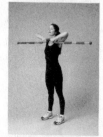
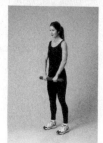
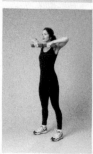

## BICEP CURL

Keep back straight, knees flexed, and feet shoulder width apart.

A. Grip Aerobic Bar, palms facing up and shoulder width apart. Hold bar with arms fully extended at front of thighs.

B. Keeping elbows stationary and wrists firm, curl bar up to chest while exhaling. Slowly extend arms and return bar to start position while inhaling.

**OR**

Keep back straight, knees flexed, and feet shoulder width apart.

A. Grip dumbbells, palms facing up and shoulder width apart. Hold dumbbells with arms fully extended at front of thighs.

B. Keeping elbows stationary and wrists firm, curl dumbbells up to chest while exhaling. Slowly extend arms and return dumbbells to start position while inhaling.

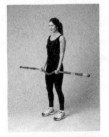
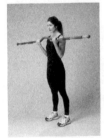
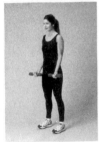
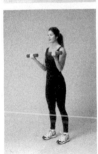

## TRICEP KICKBACKS

Keep back straight, knees flexed, and feet shoulder width apart.

A. Grip Aerobic Bar with arms fully extended at buttocks, palms facing outward.

B. Keeping elbows stationary and wrists firm, raise bar behind your buttocks as far as possible while exhaling. Keeping arms straight, lower bar to buttocks while inhaling.

### OR

Keep back straight, knees flexed, and feet shoulder width apart.

A. Grip dumbbells with arms fully extended at buttocks, palms facing outward.

B. Keeping elbows and wrists firm, raise dumbbells behind your buttocks as far as possible while exhaling. Keeping arms straight, lower dumbbells to buttocks while inhaling.

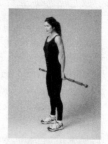

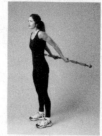

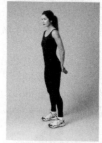

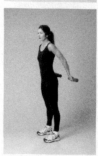

## ◆ 5. JUMPING JACKS

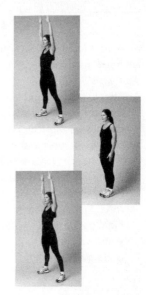

---

### JUMPING JACKS:

A. Stand with back straight, knees slightly flexed, feet wider than shoulder width apart, and arms fully extended over head.
B. Jump one inch off ground while bringing legs together and lowering arms straight to your sides.
C. Jump one inch off ground and return to starting position.

## ◆ 6. FAT BURNER

## ◆ 7. LEGS/HIPS

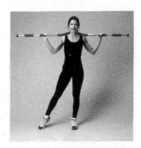

---

### STANDING KNEE TO OPPOSITE CHEST

Rest the Aerobic Bar on your neck across your shoulders, with feet shoulder width apart.

A. Transfer all weight to your left leg.
B. Raise right knee up toward your left chest to at least waist level.

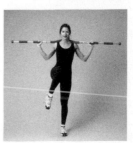

Lower right foot to starting position, touching the ground while keeping your weight on your left leg throughout the movement. Switch legs and repeat.

## L KICKS

Hold the Aerobic Bar upright with your left hand and place your right hand on your waist.

A. Start with your right leg, point your toe and gently raise your right leg straight as high as possible, without leaning your weight on bar.

B. Then touch to starting position, lightly touching the ground.

C. Pointing your toe, with leg straight, raise the right leg to the side as high as possible, without leaning your weight on bar. Switch legs and repeat.

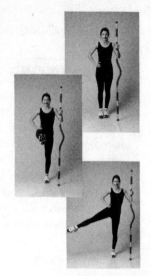

## ◆ 8. ABDOMINALS/LEGS

### SIT-UPS

**Beginner:**
Lie on back with knees bent, feet flat on the floor, fingertips on your temples. Slowly raise your head and shoulder blades off the ground. Exhale on the way up and then lower to starting position.

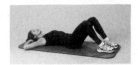
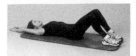

**Intermediate:**
Lie on back with knees bent, feet flat on the floor, thumbs clasped with arms extended over your head. Slowly raise your body up, bringing your chest towards your knees. Exhale while sitting up. Slowly lower body to starting position.

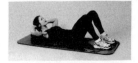
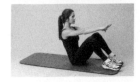

**Advanced:**
Lie on back with knees bent, feet flat on the floor, fingertips on your temples, palms facing in. Slowly raise your body up, bringing your chest towards your knees. Exhale while sitting up. Slowly lower body to starting position.

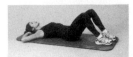
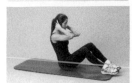

## LEG-OUTS

Lying on your back, with hands under buttocks, palms down, bring both knees in toward your chest. Slowly straighten legs out with toes pointed. Inhale while bringing knees toward chest, exhale as you straighten legs. Beginner should straighten legs out at a higher angle. As you get stronger, try to bring legs lower to the ground.

***Beginners***

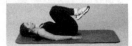

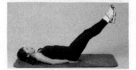

***Intermediate***

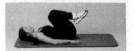

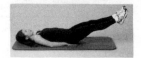

***Advanced***

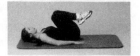

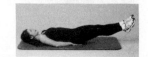

### V-SCISSORS

Lying on your back, hands at your side. Raise your legs to a 90 degree angle. While keeping back on floor, toes pointed, slowly open legs as wide apart as possible. Bring legs back together keeping toes pointed while exhaling.

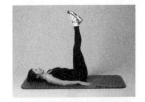

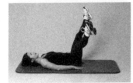

### ELBOWS-KNEES

Lying on back, raise knees and feet toward chest in a tucked position. Clasp your hands at the base of your neck. Gently curl your upper body bringing your elbows toward your knees. Slowly lower shoulders to ground. Keep lower half of your body motionless. Exhale as you bring elbows to knees.

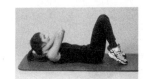

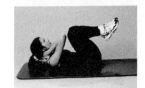

### KNEES-ELBOWS

Lying on floor, with hands clasped at the base of your neck, raise head and shoulder blades off the floor. Raise knees and feet in a tucked position toward elbows, keeping lower back pressed to the floor. Keeping tucked, lower your toes to the ground. Exhale as you raise knees to elbows.

◆ 9. FAT BURNER

◆ 10. COOL DOWN

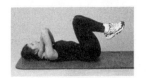

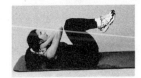

# Testimonials

As you get closer and draw nearer to your weight loss goals, keep in mind that you are building lifelong eating and exercise habits that will remain with you for many years to come. When and if you do happen to get off track with either your eating or fitness, don't despair, don't pity yourself or get disappointed with your results. Instead, put it behind you, and focus on what you need to do to get back in the game by eating sensibly and exercising regularly. Also, if you hit a plateau anytime with your weight loss goals, it's most likely because you are not exercising with enough intensity and/or you need to make adjustments with your diet in order to keep creating that deficit of calories—which is the *only* way to lose and keep weight off, whether it's 1, 10 or 50 pounds.

If you need further assistance with your weight loss objectives or have a question regarding your diet and/or exercise regimen, e-mail us at *info@exude.com* or log onto our website: *www.exude.com*. You may also call us at 1-212-644-9559 or write us at:

Exude Inc.
Attn: Program Director
16 East 52nd Street, 3rd Floor
New York, NY 10022

## ◆ TESTIMONIALS

**NAME:** Heather Passaro
**AGE:** 46
**TOTAL INCHES LOST:** 55.50
**TOTAL WEIGHT LOST:** 60+
**TIME IT TOOK TO LOSE WEIGHT:** 1 year
**PRIOR EXERCISE REGIMEN:** No prior exercise history
**APPROACH TAKEN:** Exercises 5 days per week, with moderate changes to diet

**CURRENT EXERCISE REGIMEN:** Full body routine 3 times per week for 60 minutes, including stationary biking, jumping rope, calisthenics, abdominal exercises, light weights/high repetitions for both upper and lower body. 2 times per week of aerobic exercise and abdominal exercises for 50 minutes.

**PRIOR EATING HABITS:** Heather had poor eating habits, eating too large a portion of whatever she wanted or she attempted extreme diets, but to no avail.

**CURRENT EATING HABITS:** Eats practically anything she wants, but in moderation. She is conscious, though, of limiting starchy foods, especially at night, less snacking on junk, makes healthier choices.

**THE MAIN FACTOR THAT HELPED HEATHER TO ESCAPE HER WEIGHT:** "The fact that here was another summer and I was still overweight, in fact I was very overweight and it was getting physically uncomfortable for me to do the day-to-day things—not to mention that I knew I might also be endangering my health. I wanted to look fit and healthy and then realized I would have to buy a size 18 bathing suit from the chubby girls department at Lord & Taylor! That was it; I couldn't go through the rest of my life this way. I had to fix my problem."

## ◆ BACK TO A MORE BALANCED BODY, MIND & SPIRIT: FROM HEATHER

I'm sitting at my computer and it's summer in the city. Hot, humid, sticky and irritable. I just got laid off from my job and I'm depressed; not so much about losing my job—after all this is New York City; you can always get another job. It was more about the fact that here was another summer and I was overweight, in fact I was very overweight and it was getting physically uncomfortable and I knew I might also be endangering my health.

In California where I grew up, if you have time off with unemployment benefits you do what all California girls do: you check the want ads on Sunday, mail out your résumés on Monday and wait it out for the rest of the week at the beach while working on your tan. Well, this was New York City and getting to the surf and sand is complicated and the thought of wanting to work on a tan to look fit and healthy in a size 18 bathing suit from the chubby girls department at Lord & Taylor wasn't exactly appealing! That was it; I couldn't go through the rest of my life this way. I had to fix my problem, but I couldn't do it with food. Diets had never worked for me. In fact my sister snapped on the phone "Heather, you're the worst dieter." It may have been a passing comment but something about her tone was more like a slap. I took it to mean that my friends and family don't take me seriously. I had to switch my focus off of food and find another way.

I was logging on ready to search for my next Monster Job, Hot Job or whatever job and there was this flash on my AOL home page. "Learn How Miss Universe Lost All Her Weight! Donald Trump Employs Exude Fitness in NYC to Trim Down Chubby Beauty." I'm curious and decide to give Exude a call. I didn't want to lose my focus. "Can I come in right now?" That was the first day of my journey back to a more balanced body, mind and spirit.

I shower, blow-dry my hair and do my makeup, and for what? You're going to workout silly, and it's the middle of August so you're going to look like a melted grilled cheese sandwich when you get there. I ignore myself. I head up on the subway to midtown with my workout clothes and sneakers. One of Exude's directors, Jason, puts me through a workout. "This is not a gym, it's a fitness center," he tells me. Cool! Here's my Amex. I had made a commitment of some serious $$. What was Ira, my significant other, going to say? What could he say? "Honey, I love you just the way you are." Maybe he does but modern psychology teaches us "you have to love yourself before anyone else can love you." So I explained to him it had nothing to do with money but about self-love.

When he still didn't get it, I told him my severance would just about cover it. "Fine," he said.

It's now been nearly 16 months and I have been exercising and eating healthier thanks to the commonsense approach that Exude has taught me. Aside from now being fit for the first time in my life, I look and feel 20 years younger. I am extremely healthy and fit and know that I will stick with this program for the rest of my life.

Sincerely,

Heather

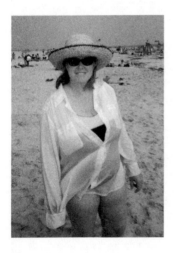
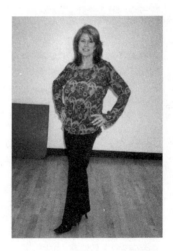

**NAME:** Nancy Hsu
**AGE:** 18
**TOTAL INCHES LOST:** 12
**TOTAL WEIGHT LOST:** 30
**TIME IT TOOK TO LOSE THE WEIGHT:** 6 months

**PRIOR EXERCISE REGIMEN:** I exercised for about 5 months without seeing major results before going to Exude. I would do 10 minutes on the elliptical, then an hour or more of 2-minute intervals between level 10 and level 2 intensity. Sometimes after that, I would hop on the bike for another 30 minutes of a cardio program. My exercise was mainly on the elliptical and it was not a very healthy exercise program as I was always there for more than two hours at a time. I didn't think I could continue doing that forever but was not sure what else to do to get results.

**APPROACH TAKEN:** Exercised 3–4 times a week, better moderation with food.

**CURRENT EXERCISE REGIMEN:** While at Exude, Nancy did an Exude moderate to advanced full body routine 4–5 times a week which included: jumping rope, calisthenics and light resistance/high repetitions for upper and lower body, abdominal exercises. Nancy has been back at school now and has accomplished one of her many goals and joined the women's rowing team. Nancy continues with her Exude workout 2–3 times a week in addition to running 4 miles a day along with other strength training/cardio, working on the ergometer and doing crew exercisers similar to calisthenics called "scullers": arms in, legs out, arms out, legs in, resting on butt, plus: **Plyos: jumpies:** jumping high up in the air and getting butt all the way down to the ground, **Mountain climbers,** (I'm sure you know what these are, hands on ground, alternating feet back and forth), **swimmers** (stomach on floor, lifting quads up back and forth 30 seconds at a time), **running stairs** once a week (40 flights, 2 steps at a time), doing **6k ergometer tests** once a week with an average split under 2 minutes and 25 seconds, as well as actually rowing in the boat.

**PRIOR EATING HABITS:** I was not very health minded or educated about what to do before I started exercising, and ate whatever and how much I wanted. When I started exercising I did the other extreme and was very restrictive, cutting out all carbohydrates and eating only grilled chicken for every meal with an occasional fruit and/or vegetable. I was not sure how to modify or increase portions without getting hungry.

**CURRENT EATING HABITS:** I make much better choices now and understand portion control and eating the right amounts of food that I know I will burn when I exercise. I typically eat a good breakfast every morning consisting of bowl of Special K with a yogurt and sometimes a banana or a small low fat bran muffin. Light lunches consist of a salad or hummus wrap and my dinner is usually steamed vegetables and a serving of pasta salad with some chickpeas. Or just another huge salad. I try to eat as little red meat as possible. I watch what snacks I eat during the day but especially after 8 P.M. My occasional snack is baked chips and once in a while Gummi bears.

**THE MAIN FACTOR THAT HELPED NANCY TO ESCAPE HER WEIGHT:** Meeting with an Exude consultant and watching what I ate without depriving myself definitely helped me achieve my goals. I had amazing support and excitement from the Exude staff when I made improvements in my workout or in my weight/inch loss which really motivated me to do better every time I did the workout.

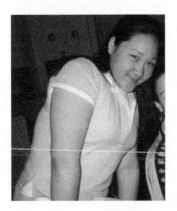
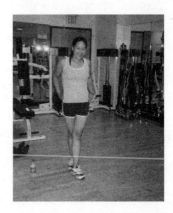

## ◆ WITHIN TWO WEEKS MY CLOTHES FIT BETTER: FROM NANCY

As my senior year of high school headed toward its end, my worries switched from college admissions to what I was going to wear to the prom. In February, I made the decision to lose weight to look great for that one night in June. My weight loss plan included working out at least 3 days a week, and consisted of an hour of cardio each day. I lost 10 pounds by June and felt great so I bought a new wardrobe to motivate myself to continue. Soon after that, I felt healthier and had more energy but no matter how much exercise I did, I was unable to lose more weight. I needed a new approach to achieving the body I wanted, and luckily came across NYC's Exude.com Fitness in a fashion magazine.

After much reading about Exude, I rewarded myself by setting up a fitness orientation at Exude with Lee Ross. I wanted to start a new life with the guidance that Exude had to offer me. I was happy to see that after only a couple of sessions with my trainer, I was stronger and more flexible. My entire workout routine was changed and adapted to fit my needs. I had specific off-day workouts to do when I was not at Exude and then wonderful challenging workouts when I was at Exude. Within 2 weeks I noticed that my clothes fit better and I was finally able to wear tiny tank tops without feeling at all self-conscious. Now it was the end of July and I had lost a total of twenty pounds!

I followed the Exude programs outlined for me throughout the rest of the summer and lost ten more pounds and a total of 12 inches and have never felt better about myself. I have never jumped rope before Exude and now consider it the best and only tool I need to be physically fit. I enjoyed every session at Exude and am going to take everything I learned with me to college. In all, I have lost a total of thirty pounds in about 6 months and I plan to lose more since now can work out the smart way and the right way for me.